THOMAS GLASS MD

Thomas Glass MD

PHYSICIAN OF GEORGIAN EXETER

Alick Cameron

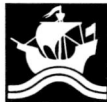

DEVON BOOKS

First published in Great Britain in 1996 by Devon Books

British Library Cataloguing in Publication Data
CIP data for this work is available from the British Library

ISBN 0 86114 906 8

DEVON BOOKS

Official Publisher to Devon County Council
Halsgrove House, Lower Moor Way
Tiverton, Devon EX16 6SS

Tel: 01884 243242
Fax: 01884 243325

Cover illustrations: The front jacket illustration is a portrait of
Thomas Glass MD, by John Opie (1761-1807) - by kind permission of the
Royal Devon & Exeter Healthcare NHS Trust. The map on the back cover is
a detail from Tozer's map of the city, published in 1792.

Printed in Great Britain by Longdunn Press Ltd, Bristol

From the facts recorded, it will be obvious, that Dr Glass's success was rather owing to a series of Events peculiarly fortunate, than to his Talents, Labour, and Assiduity. Prudence had little share in concerting or bringing them to their fortunate issue. His reserve was not impenetrable; his manners not conciliatory; and He was respected for his medical Talents, rather than admired for his general knowledge. He possessed the confidence rather than the affections of his fellow citizens: He was more respectable than amiable. His mind was indeed always of the sterner mould; harshly severe rather than mildly affectionate.

BARTHOLEMEW PARR M.D.,
Biographical Anecdotes of the late Dr Glass of Exeter, 1795.

In an obscure corner of the yard, behind the church, is interred the body of the late Dr Glass, of Exeter, whose professional skill, eminent learning, and amiable disposition, justly acquired the esteem of all his numerous acquaintance;

ALEXANDER JENKINS,
History of the City of Exeter, 1806.

DEDICATION

For Angela and Charlotte

Contents

Glassiana

... it is equally certain that many Patients, treated with the cooling Regimen, and given over, as past all Hopes of Recovery, by those under whose care they were, have been to the no small Disgrace of the Faculty, brought to life again by drinking Wine, strong Beer, or Brandy, which was given to them by some old woman, contrary to orders, until their heart was well cheared, their blood warmed, and they fell fast asleep. So many instances of this kind have happened everywhere, and are so well known, that these are sufficient to account for the favourable opinion the bulk of mankind entertain of Nurse's skill in managing the Small-pox.

First letter to Dr Baker

Mercurial powders, and gentle purges, with a strict regimen, free use of air, and moderate exercise, are very little to be depended upon for preventing a bad sort of Pox when the infection is taken in the natural way.

First letter to Dr Baker

... many people are infatuated by their prejudices for what has been long practised and generally approved. But are there not others of a quite contrary disposition, who are prevented from making a proper use of their senses and reason by an over-fondness for what is new and extraordinary?

Second letter to Dr Baker

... a Physician ought not to seize his Patient by the Hand immediately, at his first coming in, but to sit down by him, and with a cheerful Countenance, enquire how he finds himself; and if he is under any Fear of Danger, to encourage him with proper Discourse, and then feel his pulse.

Sixth Commentary, quoting *Celsus* (book III, chapter 6).

I set about reducing the matter Hippocrates has left us, under such Heads as seemed to me most convenient, one of which was of Fevers. On perusing what I had collected together, I imagined that the History and Cure of Fevers, taken from Hippocrates, would be no unacceptable Present to young Practioners: for this Distemper is the most common, and the most fatal, of all that afflict Mankind; and though some Physicians may have differed from Hippocrates as to the method of Cure, yet all allow that he was the best acquainted with the Signs of Diseases, and their Portent.

Preface to the Twelve Commentaries on Fevers.

It therefore necessarily follows, that there is no absolute vice, evil, or imperfection in the universe. And God, who surveys, and who alone can possibly survey the whole of being, and the whole of every particular being, not successively or partially, but at once, sees that every thing, which he has made, is very good, and he perfectly approves of all his works.

These conclusions, I am sensible, disagree with some doctrines, which are supposed to be contained in the scriptures; if they really are contrary to any doctrine therein contained, I am convinced they are false. But it ought to be well considered, that the scriptures, in condescension to the imperfection and narrowness of our intellectual faculties and capacities, speak for the most part the popular language, and very frequently compare heavenly or spiritual things with those which are the objects of our senses. They represent God as a man, who loves, pities, hates, repents, is provoked to anger, wrath, and revenge. And who, as an earthly father, master, judge, and king, chastises, corrects, punishes, executes vengeance, and destroys his rebellious subjects, and irreconcileable enemies. We are not therefore to believe, as some have, and do, that God really grieves, hates, repents, is angry, and takes vengeance; since it is absolutely impossible, that a being, "in whom there is no variableness, nor shadow of turning, and who is the same today, yesterday, and for ever", should be modified by human passions or affections: for then he would necessarily be a various changeable thing.

Meditation upon the Attributes of God
and the Nature of Man (page 56).

Acknowledgements

I wish particularly to express my gratitude to Mrs Ruth Wesierska, a descendant of Thomas Glass, who was herself at one time planning a book on her ancestor and who, with the utmost kindness and generosity, passed on to me the result of her research. This was especially helpful in regard to family connections. Another descendant to whom I am much indebted is the Right Honourable, the Lord Borthwick, for his courtesy in allowing me to inspect his family archive, his portrait of Thomas Glass in middle life, by Hudson, the correspondence relating to it, and Thomas Glass's MD diploma from Leyden. It is with his permission that I reproduce both portrait and diploma, photographed by Hector Innes of Kelso.

I received early encouragement from Professor Roy Porter and Professor William Bynum, of the Wellcome Institute for the History of Medicine. Both were kind enough to read the first draft, deserving my thanks. Many helpful suggestions, to a tiro stumbling where angels would only venture anxiously, were provided by Dr Jonathan Barry of the Department of History and Archaeology, University of Exeter. He also located two elusive tracts. My friend Rex Browning, whose opinion I value, also ploughed through the first draft, choking back his innate antipathy to matters medical.

I acknowledge with gratitude the information I have gleaned from P.M.G. Russell's *History of the Exeter Hospitals*; likewise I am greatly indebted to Ronald Impey for his great patience in taking me through the Latin of Thomas Glass's MD dissertation. The inadequacy of the result is due to me alone; the literal, more naive, approach was preferred to a more elegant (but perhaps less accurate) free translation.

Both West Country Studies Library staff and those in the Devon Record Office have shown me never-failing friendly co-operation, as have the librarians of Exeter Cathedral Library, the Devon and Exeter Institution, and Exeter University Library. Further afield, I owe so much to the librarians of the Royal College of Physicians, the Wellcome Institute, the Royal Society of Medicine, The Bodleian Library, the Centre for Oxfordshire Studies (Central Library, Oxford), and Dr Williams' Library, for their patience. In addition, valuable help from the archivists at Queen's College, University College, and Oriel College, Oxford, and the Worshipful Society of Apothecaries, is willingly acknowledged.

The Royal Devon and Exeter Healthcare NHS Trust have very kindly allowed reproduction of several portraits in their possession, of which the Paul Mellon Centre for Studies in British Art supplied the photographs. My long-suffering wife and daughter have put up patiently with long absences upstairs, the one convinced that my word processor had some kind of feminine charms, the other that Thomas Glass must be some sort of great grandfather.

Introduction

A number of West Country physicians achieved notoriety in one way or another in the eighteenth century: Baker and Battie settled in London, Glynn in Cambridge; Huxham and the two Musgraves remained in Devon, though Samuel, the younger one, full of such early promise, lurched off the straight path and landed eventually and uncertainly in London; William Oliver, a Cornishman, removed to Bath (why does that conjunction evoke a fleeting smile?).[1]

Another was Thomas Glass (1709-1786), a Tiverton man, who subsequently moved to Exeter where he passed all his professional life.

Thomas was the second son of Michael Glass, a dyer. As a dissenter, no rarity in that region of those days, and thus denied access to an English University, he enrolled at Leyden where he matriculated on 29 October 1728, graduating MD in July 1731.[2]

His father's death in 1732 brought Thomas back to Tiverton as sole executor of the estate; of his nine brothers and sisters four had died, including his elder brother. Samuel, next in line, had been apprenticed to Nicholas Peters, a surgeon apothecary at Topsham, since 1729,[3] and Michael, now thirteen, was due to take over the family business at the age of twenty-one.

This had to be a time of reflection and adjustment for a young man of twenty-three, suddenly, as his father's sole executor, saddled with making provision for his mother and his five brothers and sisters. He married in 1737, Mary Hodges, daughter of Sir Nathaniel Hodges.

Three years later Thomas moved to Exeter; a vacancy for a physician had arisen in 1740, on the death of the well-established Dr William Williams[4]. August 27, 1741 saw the laying of the foundation stone of the Devon and Exeter Hospital and a month later the staff were appointed, of whom Thomas Glass was one of the physicians.[5]

From then on there was no stirring from Exeter, and he applied himself assiduously to building up a reputation, which in its flowering was certainly an enviable one for a provincial physician. His lucid style and easy Latin, together with his love of books, made it inevitable that he should write, and so a number of works flowed from his pen.[6]

His principal book was published in 1742, and there were a number of editions. This was *Commentarii duodecim de febribus ad Hippocratis disciplinam accommodati (The Twelve Commentaries on Fevers)*, translated into English in 1752 by Nicholas Peters, his apothecary friend, to whom his brother Samuel had been apprenticed.

Regrettably, few documents and little personal correspondence remain which would enable the bare bones, as set out in the *Dictionary of National Biography*, to be clothed in flesh and blood. How different the story might

11

have been had some garrulous old hypochondriac such as Samuel Johnson, an almost exact contemporary, passed his life in Exeter. He is mentioned with approbation by many of his peers during his life time, appearing in the writings of such as John Huxham, Thomas Percival, William Carter, Edward Spry and Nicholas May; furthermore, apart from the customary newspaper anodyne obituaries, echoes of esteem and affection continued to appear in writing in Exeter for some seventy years from such as Polwhele, Jenkins, Oliver and Munk.

Thomas was honoured by the Royal Society of Medicine of Paris by election as an honorary associate in 1776, no mean attainment, for among others elected at this time were such lions as Pringle, Cullen, Baker, Lind, Fothergill and Heberden.[7] To mark this, it was said that Thomas, always a lover of the Antients, was preparing a new fully annotated edition of the first four books of *De Medicina* of Celsus. Hitherto the only evidence of this has been a partially annotated copy of the work amongst the valuable collection of medical books, which Thomas bequeathed to Exeter Cathedral library, though Parr,[8] in 1795, referring to three volumes of manuscript notes. These disappeared mysteriously from Exeter, but very recently were discovered to have been dormant in the Bodleian Library since 1848. Oddly, the introduction to this huge commentary was written in 1762, whereas the French honour did not come until fourteen years later, so the idea was already long in train.

The most detailed appraisal of Thomas Glass's life, however, was made in 1795 by a contemporary, Bartholemew Parr (1750-1810); this was nine years after his subject's death, and is of very considerable interest, not least in what is revealed of the character of the writer himself. Parr gave two lectures entitled 'Biographical anecdotes of the late Doctor Glass of Exeter' to A Society of Gentlemen in Exeter, founded in 1792 by Dr Hugh Downman.[8] These were subsequently lodged, duly edited, in manuscript in the library of the Royal College of Physicians. Parr had graduated MD at Edinburgh in 1773 and succeeded Glass as physician to the Devon and Exeter Hospital when he retired in 1775. His commentary merits close scrutiny but must be treated with circumspection, if not frank disbelief in parts, for he betrays in his words a deep-rooted envy of his subject which goes far beyond a portrait with all the 'roughnesses, pimples, warts and everything', cynically ignoring the honoured instruction that 'one should speak only good of the dead'. His method was sly and distasteful, one of damning with faint praise; a grudging acknowledgement of some achievement, followed by a spiteful denigration; the serpent under the innocent flower. There is an irony in the motto, borrowed from Horace, with which Parr adorned his first lecture:

> ... *et incedis per ignes*
> *suppositos cineri doloso.*
> (... *and thou art walking, as it were, over fires*
> *hidden beneath treacherous ashes).*[9]

One may speculate on Hugh Downman's opinion of this account, so much at variance with the sentiments expressed in his sonnet to Dr Glass, published retrospectively in 1792:

Glass, who thy proper dignity of soul
Consulting, independently has run
The race of reason, scorning the controul
Of vulgar prejudice, nor ever won
To humour fools; rejecting little arts
Which often subjugate inferior hearts.
Having to learning, long experience joined,
From dry antiquity's obscurer store
The brighter portion culled, and well refined
The mass confused with all of modern lore;
Adapting physic to the truest scale
Which human nature can; what curious tale
Shall I devise, for sending rhimes to thee?
And yet, not sent, would my own mind be free?[10]

Three years before his death, the Medical Society at Exeter sought Thomas's agreement to having his portrait painted by Opie,[11] thus paying him a unique compliment. This was duly done and placed in the boardroom of the hospital, the following inscription being placed below:

May it be remembered that
Thomas Glass M.D.
introduced into this city and neighbourhood a method of treating
continual fevers without inflammation, by which they are rendered less
grievous, lasting, and destructive, and the miliary fever which was in
those parts a common, tedious, and fatal disease has been almost totally
extinguished, so that it now seldom occurs and when it does is soon
over.

To express their grateful sense of this and other advantages which the
Public has received from the long and extensive Practice and the
learned and judicious writings of their worthy fellow citizen, the
Medical Faculty of Exeter have placed his portrait in this Hospital, of
which he was one of the physicians thirty years.[12]

Further evidence of the approval of the majority of his colleagues is indicated by his election as President of the Hospital on March 17, 1785, the only medical man ever to hold this office; he was not destined to live out his full year of the presidency, dying on February 5, 1786.

Gordon Goodwin, in his assessment in the *Dictionary of National Biography*, stated that Glass was considered the greatest English authority, after Sir William Watson, on inoculation for the smallpox;[13] this could no doubt be disputed. His two long published letters to Dr (later Sir George) Baker[13] are of particular interest, being objective and nonpropagandist. The papers of Watson and Glass concerning inoculation were jointly translated into German. Amongst Thomas's other writings were *An Account of the Antient Baths and their Uses in Physic*, in 1752, and a pamphlet entitled *An Examination of Mr. Henry's Strictures on Glass's Magnesia*, in 1774 (a defence of his late brother's process of making *Magnesia Alba*, against some eighteenth century industrial piracy). Lastly John Fothergill asked him to contribute 'An Account of the Influenza, as it appeared at Exeter in 1775' to *Medical Observations and Inquiries*.[14]

There were two more works, not of a medical nature, which appeared in 1770 and 1772. They were published anonymously, the first *Meditations upon the Attributes of God, and the Nature of Man*. The second was *A View of Revealed Religion, as it stands to the Reason*.[15]

At a distance of two centuries, there is little enough on which to base a closeup of the real Thomas Glass. The discordant counterpoint provided by Bartholemew Parr opposes enigmatically the prevailing opinion of his worth. Questions pose themselves: what horsepower was his internal engine? Did he like a good tune, a well-turned rhyme, or a comely leg? The few of his letters that remain are on subjects that provide no such revelation, nor whether his serious professional persona was leavened by a twinkle now and then. There is little doubt that he was jealous of his reputation and was deeply touched by that gesture of his colleagues, remembering each one with a mourning ring at his death, and leaving for medical posterity his most important library, indeed a monument more valuable, if not more lasting, than brass.

On the basis that an individual shows something of himself when he writes, as much of his best-known book as can conveniently be handled, is included in chapter four. Rather than attempt a synopsis it seemed preferable to retain the eighteenth-century flavour by quoting a number of short passages from the original. Being prompted by curiosity to unravel the content of his MD dissertation, the resulting clumsy translation is included as an appendix.

It seems from his published work that Glass was suspicious of the medical 'systems' that cropped up periodically in the eighteenth century;[16] Hoffman gets an occasional nod, usually in connection with some uncontentious clinical point, but he seldom, if ever, refers to Stahl; yet either eclecticism or bibliophily led him to include three books by the former and four by the latter in his extensive medical library; in this sense he was a traditionalist, the systematists muddied the waters without any very obvious gain; so it was safer to carry the banner of the Antients, to return to the starting point, hence the theme in his 'Twelve commentaries on fevers accommodated to the teaching of Hippocrates'. One feels that insofar as Boerhaave was both his mentor and hero, he was less than enthusiastic that the great man had felt that

Hippocratism was not enough; consequently he had been moved to introduce his concept of viscidity and 'lentor'. Andrew Cunningham has suggested that Boerhaave achieved a personal reconciliation by taking to Hippocrates certain attitudes from his own day;[17] be that as it may, it seems that Boerhaave's eirenic attitude[18] rubbed off on Glass and that this quality appears in his writing and in the perception that fair-minded people had of him. Glass was not an innovator and perhaps in an age of enlightenment historians might find this a cause for unenthusiasm, but he was a thoughtful and bookish man who espoused new ideas (such as smallpox inoculation) with energy and enthusiasm.

John Opie, in his portrait, shows a benign, bewigged figure with the red cloak and gold-headed cane of the physician. The expression is calm, relaxed, but with that hint of mobility of the features that could with provocation break into a smile, even a faintly mischievous one.

Notes

ABBREVIATIONS TO NOTES THROUGHOUT:
DRO - DEVON RECORD OFFICE
DNB - DICTIONARY OF NATIONAL BIOGRAPHY
TDA - TRANSACTIONS OF THE DEVONSHIRE ASSOCIATION

(1) Sir George Baker (1722-1809), became a royal physician and president of the Royal College of Physicians; William Battie, like him, was born at Modbury, in 1704, a pioneer in the treatment of mental illness, he became President of the Royal College of Physicians in 1764, having been elected F.R.S. in 1741. Robert Glynn (1719-1800), born near Bodmin, was a fellow of King's College, passing almost the whole of his professional life at Cambridge. William Musgrave F.R.S. (1655-1721), author of *De Arthritide Symptomatica*, etc., physician at Exeter. Samuel Musgrave (1732-1780), scholar and sometime physician at Exeter (greatnephew of the former). John Huxham F.R.S. (1672-1768), author and physician at Plymouth. William Oliver F.R.S. (1695-1764), father in law of Sir John Pringle, inventor of the biscuit and physician at Bath. There was another William Oliver F.R.S. (1659-1716), a Cornishman; the main part of his life, full of excitement, was passed as a a military surgeon and then as a Physician in the Royal Navy. He divided his time between London and Bath and was latterly physician to the Royal Hospital at Greenwich.

(2) Archives of the University of Leyden, ASF 14, p. 41 and ASF 415, p. 300.

(3) See P.J. and R.V. Wallis, *Eighteenth Century Medics*, (Newcastle, 1988).

(4) Alexander Jenkins, *History of the City of Exeter and its Environs*, (Exeter, 1806), p.428. Description of memorial tablet. Wallis, op. cit. incorrectly gives date of death as 1735.

(5) J. Delpratt Harris, *The Royal Devon and Exeter Hospital* (Exeter, 1922) pp. 10,11.

(6) Professor R.S.Speck, *Doctor Glass of Exeter*, Paper read before the Bay Area History of Medicine Club on March 13, 1974. Reviewing the Glass collection in Exeter

Cathedral library he said: 'I have to believe that there was a little of the bibliomaniac in old Dr Glass. Why else have the magnificent Venice incunabulum edition of Celsus when he had three other sets of that text?'

(7) See *Medical and Philosophical Commentaries*, 1776, p. 348.

(8) This was also known as The Literary Society of Exeter. Its members took it in turns to deliver papers on a wide range of interests. They included Polwhele, Kendall, Sheldon, the surgeon and anatomist, and, for a time, Isaac d'Israeli. The Devon and Exeter Institution has a volume of their published lectures (1796).

(9) Horace, *Odes*, Book II, Ode I, line 7. The translation is by C.E. Bennet, (Loeb Classical Library).

(10) Hugh Downman, MD, *Poems to Thespia*. (Exeter, 1792). p.142.

(11) John Opie, R.A. (1761-1807)

(12) The portrait now hangs in the Post Graduate centre of the Royal Devon and Exeter Hospital, the modern successor to the original hospital. See P.M.G.Russell, *A History of the Exeter Hospitals*, (Exeter, 1976), p.41.

(13) *A letter... to Dr Baker on the means of procuring a distinct and favourable kind of smallpox*, (London, 1767). And *A second letter ... to Dr Baker on certain methods of treating the smallpox during the eruptive state*, (London, 1767). The two letters are 72 and 55 pages, respectively.

(14) *Medical Observations and Inquiries*, (London, 1784), VI, p.364. A Medical Society had been founded in London by John Fothergill in 1752, which produced six volumes of these medical essays. See R. Hingston Fox, *Dr John Fothergill and his Friends* (London, 1919), p. 141.

(15) The first of these two tracts was published in London (printed for B. Law and B. Thorne, Exeter); there are copies in the National Library of Scotland and the British Library. (ESTC.172005) The second, also published in London (printed for and sold by B. Law; Howes, Clarke and Collins; and B. Thorne, Exeter. Copies are in Cambridge University Library and Dr Williams Library. (ESTC.t177129) They are of 72 pages, octavo, and 198 pages respectively.

(16) See Andrew Cunningham, 'Boerhaave's medical system' in A. Cunningham and R. French (eds.), *The medical enlightenment of the eighteenth century* (Cambridge,1990), p. 42.

(17) *Ibid.*, p. 49.

(18) *Ibid.*, p. 48.

CHAPTER I

Tiverton, Leyden,
and the Move to Exeter

When Michael Glass died in 1732 his father, Thomas senior, was still alive. Thomas junior's great grandfather, also Michael, and a dyer in the family tradition, had an unpleasant experience during the civil war, in 1645; he narrowly escaped being shot, while sitting at his back door, on the banks of the Exe, during the siege of Tiverton Castle by the army of Fairfax.[1] Much of the prosperity of Tiverton and indeed of much of nearby Devon, revolved around the wool and cloth industry. Since the turn of the sixteenth century the Devon cloth industry had been booming. From the purely industrial standpoint, Tiverton may even have outranked Exeter.[2] The ancillary trades such as dying and fulling thrived on the coat-tails of wool, and the Glass family evidently reaped the benefit, as witness the property itemised in their wills and marriage settlements.[3] Risdon in 1608, describing Tiverton, said: 'The town is full of people, and inhabited by rich clothiers.'[4]

The Glasses were Baptists, but in 1687 an independent sect of Baptists had been founded in the town by the Rev. John Moore, recently arrived from Suffolk. To him the family remained faithful until his death in 1739.[5] Strangely, one may think, in 1702 Thomas Glass senior was made a church-warden of Tiverton, despite his dissenting status, an office which held responsibilities for the poor of the parish.[6]

The Rev. John Moore presided over a school in Peter Street and gave the young Thomas Glass his early education. Later, Thomas came under the tutelage of André de Majendie, a Huguenot emigré, one of many who had settled in Exeter after the revocation of the edict of Nantes in 1685. St Olave's church in Fore Street, Exeter, had been lent to the community, which included a school.[7]

Mary Hodges, who married Thomas on February 10, 1737 was a Londoner; her father, Sir Nathaniel, had been a Deputy Lieutenant of Middlesex and Colonel of the 2nd Regiment of Tower Hamlets. He was knighted by George I when he led a deputation to him in 1727, to present a humble address from the Deputy Lieutenants. The wedding took place at the French Protestant Church of St Martin Orgars, thus perhaps showing the Huguenot influence and a divergence from the strong Baptist tradition of both families. Sir Nathaniel, born at Taunton, was a leading Baptist minister, though he resigned in 1721; it seems that there may have been some religious disagreement, for Lady Hodges had his memorial placed in an Anglican churchyard at Stepney. She had been a Mary Buttall of Plymouth.[8]

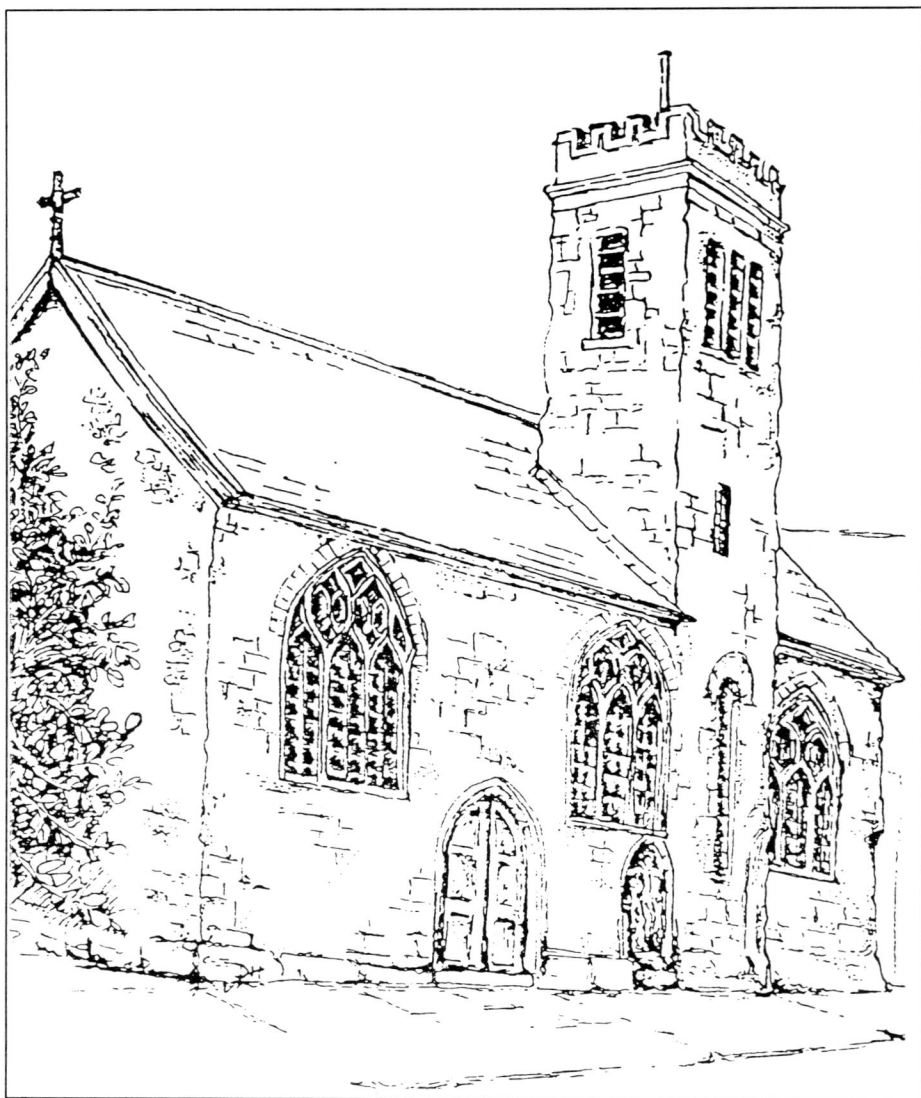

St Olave's Church, Fore Street, Exeter. Allocated to the Huguenots of Exeter 1635-1758 (reproduced by kind permission of Doreen Hatt).

Following the wedding, Thomas, now 27, and Mary went to live at the castle at Tiverton. It had a commanding view of the River and of the family home on the west bank, at West Exe. Damaged in the Civil War, the remains of the castle had been bought by Peter West, a rich wool merchant, who built a new wing in the courtyard.

18

Thomas was made Deputy Governor of Tiverton Hospital in 1738; this was the workhouse, built forty years before, to house three hundred people, and no medical duties were involved. The governors were appointed for one year from among reputable families; his father had been Treasurer in 1726.[9]

Apart from its prosperity, Tiverton was no different from any other small town in the eighteenth century. It was accepted that the hovels of the poor were warrens of filth, squalor and disease and that household refuse was automatically ejected on to the street. Smallpox hit them hard, at intervals, and typhus, typhoid, dysentery and tuberculosis carried away their victims at all times, affecting even the well-to-do, so that Michael Glass had lost four of his ten children by the time he himself died at the age of 47. Less familiar epidemics periodically swept town and country, Horace Walpole wrote on March 11, 1748:

> I have nothing to tell you but illnesses and distempers: there is what they call a miliary fever raging, which has taken off a great many people. It was scarce known till within these seven or eight years, but apparently increases every spring and autumn. They don't know how to treat it but think that they have discovered that bleeding is bad for it.[10]

Tiverton too had been periodically devasted by disastrous fires, the most recent having been in 1731.

When Thomas enrolled at Leyden in 1728, at the age of 19, he found himself amongst many compatriots; 29 English students, and 27 Scots; amongst the

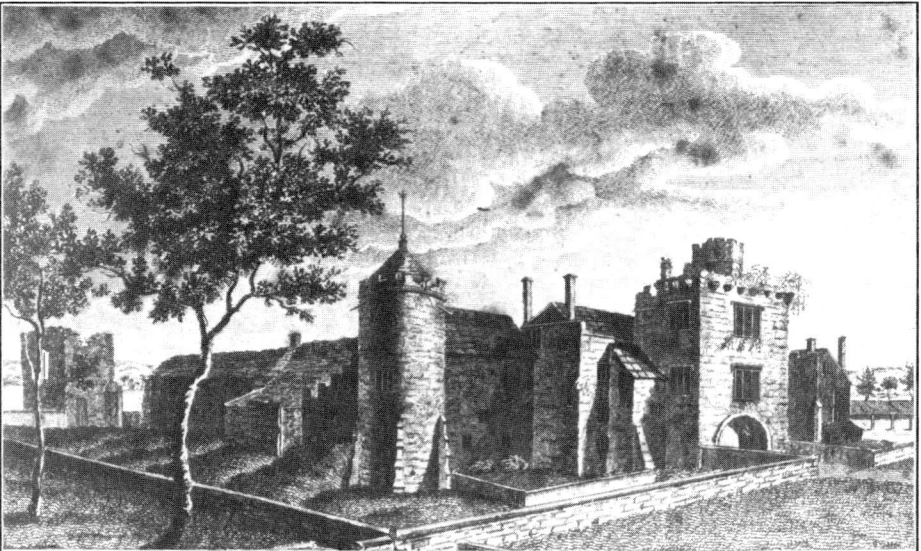

Tiverton Castle, 1730.

19

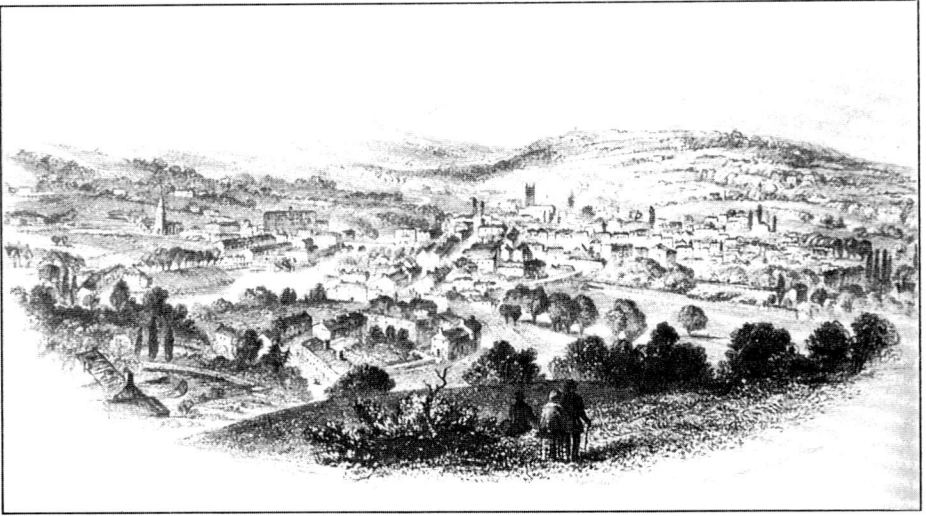

Tiverton, 1834.

former, in the faculty of letters, was Henry Fielding, and the latter included the young John Pringle, in the medical faculty. Later Thomas was to speak of Van Swieten and de Gorter as his early friends.[11]

Albinus and Gaubius were two of his teachers, but he succumbed rapidly to the spell of Boerhaave, though he was not in fact one of Boerhaave's promovendi;[12] Parr described it as blind admiration and took the opportunity of having a swipe at Boerhaave, for good measure: '... a systematic Eclectic, who had seen little practice, and was himself the Enthusiast of Hippocrates.'

It was regrettable, in Parr's eyes: '... as it led Dr Glass to undervalue the extensive Erudition of Hoffmann, the singular ingenuity and precision of Stahl.'

Bartholemew Parr may perhaps have been correct when he said that Thomas had practised medicine unsuccessfully during these years at Tiverton; Parr had consulted Elizabeth Glass, Thomas's surviving sister, according to the end-notes to his manuscript, and a certain Mr J. Smith. He pointed out with some plausibility that the practice of a profession seldom succeeds among those with whom the practitioner has lived in his early youth, but added gratuitously:

> *His manner was unpleasing, his address forbidding, and his appearance mean. When he spoke, it was with a sneer; and when he seemed to unbend, his relaxation appeared a condescension.*

It seems certain that part, at any rate, of his time at Tiverton passed in planning and writing the *Twelve Commentaries on Fevers*, to be published in 1742, in Latin, as a curtain raiser to his professional life at Exeter. Latin was

20

still very much the *lingua franca* of the academic world and at Leyden all lectures, tutorials, and examinations were conducted in it. A number of Boerhaave's textbooks, which had belonged to Thomas, have neat marginal annotations in Latin, almost certainly having been used as a concomitant to the lectures. By 1740 when Thomas and Mary moved to Exeter nine years had gone by; nine years since graduation at Leyden and the successful defence of his inaugural dissertation.[13] The aura of the magnificent Boerhaave remained with him.

Several of the Exeter physicians had either graduated at Leyden or had spent time there. Oxford and Cambridge, open only to members of the established church, provided protracted instruction in the medical classics, medical degrees, but no clinical training; their graduates either went abroad to the Continent or north to Edinburgh, already renowned, deeply influenced by Leyden and about to become the premier medical school of Europe. Michael Lee Dicker, for instance, a Quaker, had graduated MD at Leyden in 1718; he was appointed physician to the Devon and Exeter Hospital at its inception and died in office in 1751; described as:

> *a man of inoffensive manners and plain good sense, rather safe than scientific, and more distinguished for mild attention than officious interference in the operations of nature.*

These words are from *Munk's Roll*,[14] but they are also those of Bartholemew Parr, who added that he was often the subject of the coarsest and most illiberal raillery, mainly because in his youth he had been apprenticed to his uncle, who had, with some other menial occupations, practised farriery. His portrait was painted by Hudson and hangs in the boardroom of the modern hospital.

William Hallett (1693-1754) was a Leyden MD, a dissenter, and said to be implicitly trusted by those of his own persuasion in and around Exeter and another of the first six physicians at the Hospital.[15]

Brookes[16] mentions Hallet in connection with hydrophobia:

> *...many terrible Symptoms ensued, which occasioned great trouble. These Dr Nugent judged to be hysterical, and were at length cured by the following powder, which Dr Hallett of Exeter has found to be of excellent Use in some hysteric cases...*

The most significant of Thomas Glass's colleagues was John Andrew (1708-1772), born at Probus, he was a Fellow of Exeter College, Oxford, from 1733-1744, MB1739, MD 1742. He was given permission by his patron (Lord Petre) to travel abroad and in 1735 enrolled at Leyden as a student, but did not graduate there. His social standing and no doubt his career, were improved by marrying into the aristocracy, Isabella, the fifth daughter of Sir William Courtenay. Andrew was one of the first to introduce smallpox inoculation into Devon and no doubt was an influence on Glass in this respect. In 1765 he published a tract on *The Practice of Inoculation impartially considered ...* in the form of a letter to Sir Edward Wilmot. In a postscript he relates how he was requested to visit two children on the thirteenth day after inoculation, finding them both ill of the confluent smallpox. He continues:

> *From the second of June, I had no particular Account of them, till the 6th, when I visited them with my Friend and Colleague Dr Glass, which was the only Visit we made to the youngest, for he died in the Evening of the following Day; but we were desired to attend the eldest again, on the 8th, at which Time there appeared Hopes of his Recovery; and favourable Accounts of him were sent to us, till the 14th, when we were acquainted that he had brought off six Worms the Day before, and that he was in the last Extremity.*
>
> *As neither Dr Glass, nor myself, ever saw such a malignant Sort of SmallPox from inoculation, among near a thousand that have been inoculated under the Directions of one, or other, of us, as it resembled exactly the virulent Kind, which has greatly prevailed during the last six Months; and as these Children had been almost surrounded by the SmallPox, it may not, perhaps, be unjust to suppose, that the Natural Infection had reached them.*[17]

All, therefore, seems to have been cordial between Andrew and Glass, but a number of published tracts[18] indicate that Andrew had a disputacious nature and quarrelled on non-medical matters with Messrs Pitfield, Chapple and Tremlett. Andrew also was in dispute with 'An Apothecary', who, in this case was Nicholas Peters, Thomas's friend from Topsham and Cullompton to whom his brother, Samuel, had been apprenticed. Peters published his side of the matter, entitled *Observations on the state of the dispute between a physician and an apothecary, concerning a prescription of Sydenham...etc.*[19] A copy of this is among the books which belonged to Glass and bequeathed to Exeter Cathedral Library; a manuscript note against a reference to an 'experienced physician' on page 17 reads 'Dr Glass'. Peters put forward a carefully argued case against the often held view that Sydenham was incapable of writing his works in Latin.[20] He continued, quoting reputable sources, that Sydenham's dosage had been correct and safe.

It is of interest that Parr, in a mood of unusual benevolence on this matter, speaks highly, even affectionately of Peters, even giving Glass a subdued murmur of approval:

> *... a dispute occurred between a Physician and an Apothecary, Dr Andrew and Mr. Peters of Topsham, respecting a supposed Error of the Press, in a prescription of Sydenham. The Dose seemed so enormous, that it was proper to consider the subject at length. Mr. Peters' Pamphlett was written with great Candour and moderation; with much good sense and practical knowledge. He certainly was assisted,*

*in it, by Dr Glass, and I mean not to depreciate his own merit, by the
observation. He had some years before translated the Commentaries,
and I can assert that from my own knowledge that the translation was
not, as Malevolence has suggested, the English Copy which Mr. Wood
had adorned with the Roman toga.[21] Mr. Peters as Apothecary at
Topsham deserved to have been known in a more extensive sphere. He
was a good classical Scholar, an experienced, practical Chemist, and a
correct, comprehensive Philosopher. He drew with accuracy and
elegance; his conversation was lively, and his Humour facetious. It
gives me pleasure to record these traits of a man, to whom I was greatly
indebted; whose merit and good Humour enlivened many of my boyish
Hours; whose Friendship and assistance were of essential service, at
another Period. That part of his Essay, which contained a defence of
Sydenham's Scholarship, and one of the Cases, he was probably
indebted for to Dr Glass.*

John Andrew's portrait by Hudson was recently acquired by a medical group
in Exeter and is displayed in the elegant boardroom of the old hospital, now
used for administrative offices. He was friend to Dean Alured Clarke,
moving spirit behind the building of the Devon and Exeter Hospital; he was
also his physician and among the first to be appointed to the medical staff. It
was said of him that:

*he was a man of learning, polished address, unremitting in his profes-
sional exertions and at once popular with all those with whom he came
in contact.[22]*

His daughter Frances married the charming, literary, but not very robust Dr
Hugh Downman, himself in due course a member of the hospital staff.

The year after Thomas and Mary Glass arrived in Exeter the topic of hospitals
came to dominate the medical scene.

George Oliver[23] drew attention to the gross disregard of sanitary provisions
in Exeter at that time and in its train the prevalence of such diseases as gaol
fever; the only thought was of trade: 'O cives, cives, quaerenda pecunia
primum!'

Into this arena in January, 1741, came Dr Alured Clarke, formerly
Prebendary of Winchester and Westminster. He had already, in 1736, founded
a noble Public Hospital at Winchester 'for the benefit of the sick poor'. Now,
as the new Dean of Exeter, he determined:

*not to give sleep to his eyes, nor slumber to his eyelids, until he had
secured the same blessings for the County of Devon and its
Metropolis[24].*

He immediately set about canvassing subscribers to the new Devon and
Exeter Hospital, which drew an instant response from people of substance in

the area. The first General Meeting of subscribers was on July 23, 1741, the Dean taking the chair. One of the principal items discussed was the purchase of a suitable piece of land on which to build the hospital, for which an advisory subcommittee was appointed. The advantage of having an existing building which could be adapted was evident, and with this in mind Dean Clarke had applied to the City Chamber for the land and buildings of the old and dilapidated workhouse or bridewell at the lower end of Paris Street. At a meeting of the Chamber on June 29:

> *Mr Mayor acquainted this Body that he had been applied to by Mr Dean to have the present Bridewell granted to proper persons for the carrying on his intended design of erecting a Hospital. Which this Body, taking into consideration, it is Resolved that it will be highly inconvenient for this Body to part with the said House and therefore cannot comply with the Dean's Request and Mr President Blake [and others named] are desired to wait upon the Dean with the Resolution.*[25]

It may be that the civic authorities were stung because they were being shown to have been laggardly in the matter of hospitals, and decided to obstruct the outsider. It may also have been that as it had been proposed that Dean Clarke's hospital was to serve the county as well as the city, as guardians of the municipal monies, they considered that these should be spent specifically on city welfare rather than for that of the county of Devon. At all events, at a meeting of the Chamber on August 25:

> *Mr Alderman Tripe moved that the Question might be put whether the Charity intended to be bestowed by this Body should be applied for the promoting the intended Hospital, commonly called the Dean's Hospital, or whether the same should be applied to an Hospital to be set up for the Poor of this City only. The Question was put accordingly and this Body does resolve that this intended Charity be applied for the Relief of the Poor of this City only.*
> *And Mr Alderman Coplestone [and others named] or any four of them are appointed a committee to look out a proper place for the new intended Hospital and to consider what method to carry on ye said Charity.*[26]

This resolution of the Chamber is important when considering the bitter rivalry that developed subsequently between the two hospitals and emphasises that at this time the workhouse contained no significant hospital element. There were evidently also divided loyalties, for many of those attending the first meeting of subscribers to the Dean's hospital were members of the Chamber, some were aldermen, frequently maintaining their support through the troubled times ahead. Benjamin Heath, though never a member of the Chamber and not yet Town Clerk, was elected Treasurer. On reflection, perhaps out of feeling for his brother, Thomas, he sent in his resignation to the Dean on August 11; curiously the then mayor, Nicholas Lee, was elected in his place.[27]

The Dean was not one to be discouraged by the Chamber's rebuff or to let the grass grow under his feet. John Tuckfield, later to be Tory MP for the city, presented a large building site at Southernhay.[28] The money flooded in, everyone it seemed wanted to be a governor. Thousands of spectators turned up on August 27, 1741, for the laying of the foundation stone; as the *Gentleman's Magazine* for September, 1741, has it:

> *A very great Number of Gentlemen of every Party, Benefactors to the Hospital, met together at the Chapter House of St Peter, from whence they walk'd in solemn Procession, attended by the City Musick, to Southernhay, where a Party of Soldiers was drawn up, who favoured them with Three Volleys of Small Arms ... There were several Thousand People, who had the pleasure of seeing the Solemnity, and there was not one Murmur heard. Every Heart was full of Joy, too great to be express'd, and which can be imagin'd only by those who delight in the Happiness of their Fellow Creatures. The Air was filled with the Universal Shouts of the Multitude. The Rich rejoiced exceedingly that they were to be the happy Instruments of so great a Blessing to their Country, and the Poor echo'd back their Acclamations of Joy with Blessings upon their Pious and Generous Benefactors. Such a Day of Gladness has not been known here for many years..*

This certainly acted as a spur, for on September 1 the minutes of the Chamber recorded:

> *Mr Mayor producing to this Body proposals for establishing an Exeter Hospital, the same being publicly read, this Body do agree that the same be carried into Execution. £250 was allocated for this purpose, and the said proposals were ordered to be printed.*[29]

Two physicians were appointed to the City Hospital. These were Dr John Jagoe (1699-1748) and Dr George Bent (1702-1771). Jagoe had graduated MD at Exeter College, Oxford, and, although he died two years before Bartholemew Parr was born, the latter had confidence enough to state that: 'he was a man of pompous manners, proud of an English degree, and jealous of foreign graduates.'

Dr Bent had a Cambridge degree, was a product of St Catherine's College, and had previously practised at Crediton. Parr mentions that he had been distinguished as an author in the Medical Essays of Edinburgh. Unaware that the City Hospital would not survive the fierce competition, Bent found that he had backed a loser and, although he applied, was barred from appointment to a post at the new hospital; he was unable to gain a foothold there until the death of Dr Hallett in 1754, when he was 52 years old. John Andrew, his junior, overtook him and could not be dislodged; poor Bent lost the practice he had once possessed and was for some time before his death confined to his house, by increasing age and infirmities.

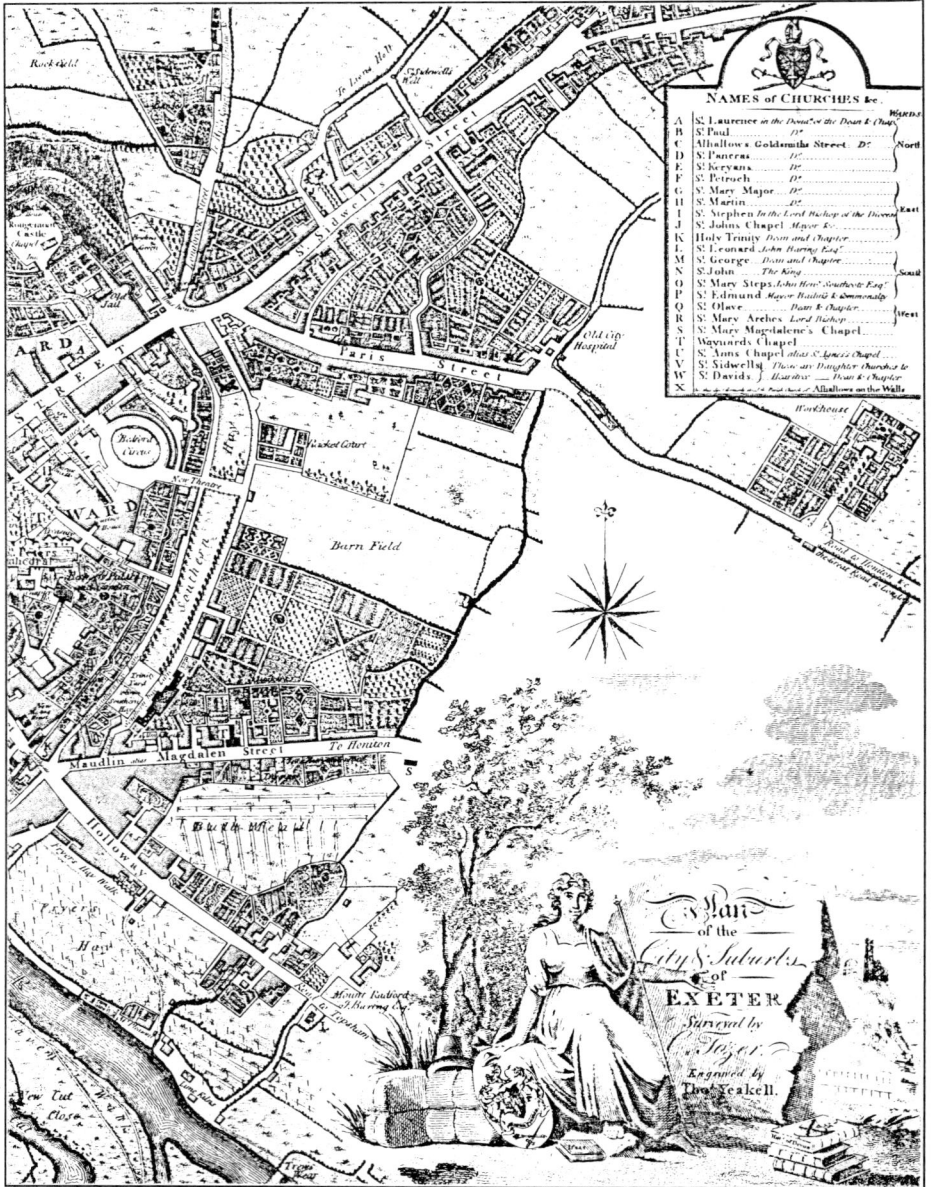

Tozer's map of Exeter, 1792, showing site of City Hospital to west of Paris Street (by kind permission of Exeter Central Library).

Surgeons to the City Hospital were John Drake and the barber-surgeon Henry Walker.[30]

Benjamin Heath, who became Town Clerk of Exeter in 1752, and Alderman Thomas Heath, his brother, mayor in 1738 and 1749, were old and valued friends of Thomas Glass; they strenuously urged his acceptance of the office of physician at the City Hospital, but he was of the opinion that their institution was not firmly established and begged their leave to decline it, in favour of the other.[31]

The Devon and Exeter Hospital made rapid strides; the City Chamber on the one hand and Church and gentry on the other, adopted embattled positions.

The honorary medical and surgical staff were elected in September, 1741. Four of the five physicians have been mentioned; the fifth was Dr Edmond Walrond (1700-1758), graduate of Balliol College, a mysterious, almost invisible person, son of Edmond Walrond of Seaton.

Of the surgeons, there were elected Bartholemew Parr senior (his physician son was not born until 1750), the Patches (father and son), Mr Pillett and Mr Walker. The latter was disqualified as, like Dr Bent, he had already signed on with the City Hospital. The resident apothecary was Mr. Lucraft.[32]

The City Hospital, already having a structure on which to work, and doubtless looking over its shoulder, also forged ahead. The City Receiver's vouchers for 1741-42 reflect a constant succession of work done or goods and materials supplied. Particularly one may note an invoice from the printer Felix Farley for 1741; here is noted: 'Printing 1500 proposals for the Exeter Hospital £4.5.0 (undated). Advertising City Hospital and Infirmary £0.3.6 (7th May, 1741).[33] The latter anticipating the first official discussions in the Chamber.

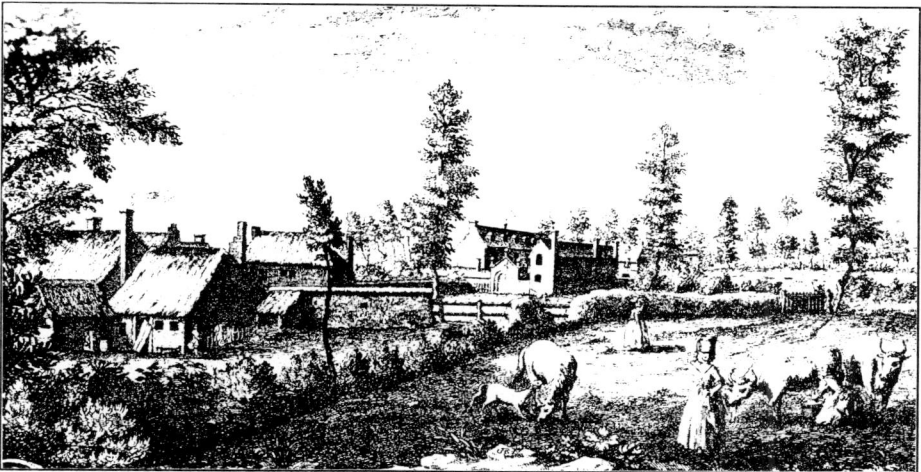

City Hospital, 1744 (by kind permission of Exeter Central Library).

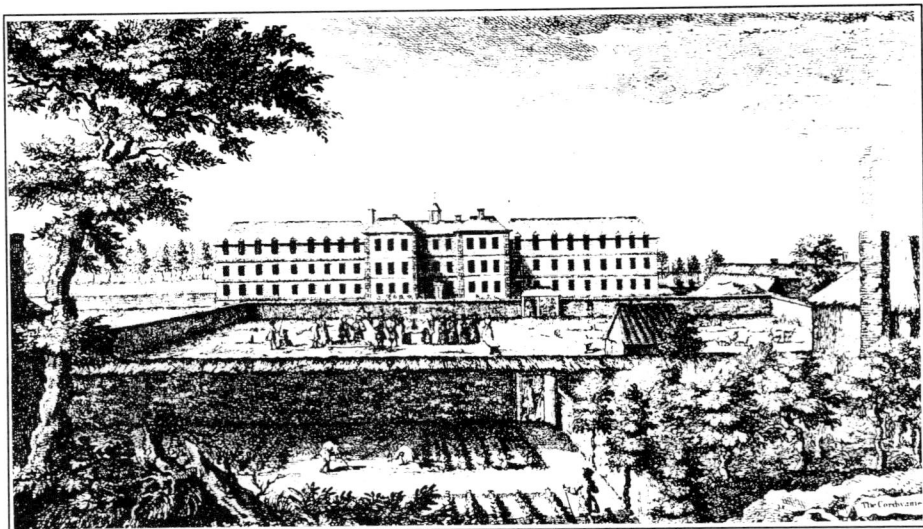

Devon and Exeter Hospital, 1744 (by kind permission of Exeter Central Library).

In the event it opened its doors, with 30 beds, four months before the Devon and Exeter Hospital declared itself open, on January 1, 1743. Dean Clarke had died on May 31, 1742, at the age of 46, so did not witness the fruition of his labours; he was buried in Westminster Abbey.

The contest between the rival hospitals continued with unabated rancour; operations and cures, performed and completed in each, were, like modern-day football results, published weekly:

> *in a plan of Exeter published under the auspices of the Chamber [Roque's map, 1744], the view of their favourite institution is adorned with a prospect of fields, and a dairymaid milking a cow, while the churchyard in front of the County Hospital, displays a funeral procession: as if one was the source of health, the other, the shortest path to the grave. Allegedly this was by no means accidental.*[34]

The City Hospital gradually dropped out of the race, its life has been reported as being about four years, but it was not until October 31, 1752 that it was finally put to rest:

> *Resolved that, from the 17th day of November next, the Exeter Hospital be no longer kept up or continued and that all the Servants of the House be at that time discharged and that no more patients be taken in from this day...*[35]

28

Notes

(1)   Bartholemew Parr, *Biographical anecdotes of the late Doctor Glass of Exeter* (1795), MS, Library of the Royal College of Physicians. Hereafter Parr.

(2)   Robert Newton, *Eighteenth Century Exeter*, (Exeter, 1984), p. 10.

(3)   Devon Record Office; will of Michael Glass, the elder, 1702 (Ref. 49/9/6/211 a); marriage settlement of Michael Glass and Elizabeth Handford, 1706 (Ref. 49/9/6/195).

(4)   Tristram Risdon, *The Chorographic description or Survey of the County of Devon*. (London, 1811) p.71. The comments were made in 1608, though not published until 1714.

(5)   Martin Dunsford, *Historical Memoirs of the Town and Parish of Tiverton*, (Exeter,1790), 2nd edition, p. 317.

(6)   *Ibid*. p. 444.

(7)   Parr, *passim*. See also Dunsford, *op. cit.* p.380.

(8)   The Baptist Historical Society records show that Sir Nathaniel Hodges was born in 1675 and became a pastor of a Baptist church in 1698. He moved to London in 1707 to take charge of the newly formed church in Artillery Lane, Spitalfields. His wife had been a Mary Buttall of Plymouth; the Devon Record Office is a source of some information about the Buttall family, in connection with the deeds of the Sugar House, to be referred to later (Ref. DD 100260). Mary was either daughter or granddaughter of Samuel Buttall, a sugar baker of Plymouth, who built the Sugar House at Topsham. A Samuel Buttall was minister of the George Street Baptist Church from 1690-1697 and was succeeded by Nathaniel Hodges from 1698-1701. It seems very likely that the two Samuels were the same. See C.W. Bracken, *History of Plymouth*, (Plymouth, 1931), p.297.

(9)   Dunsford, *op. cit.* p. 458. A footnote describes Thomas Glass as 'a very eminent physician. He was a native of Tiverton ... At the time he held the above office he resided in the new apartments of the Castle of Tiverton: from thence he went to Exon: and continued in great and respectable practice in that city a long course of years.'

(10)   Horace Walpole, *Letters to Sir Horace Mann* (Philadelphia, 1842), I, p. 545. See *Twelve Commentaries*, chapter four.

(11)   Parr, *passim*. Baron Gerhard van Swieten (1700-1772), after completing his studies at Leyden, remained there to teach, eventually moving to Vienna to resurrect the medical school there. There were two de Gorters, father and son; the former had graduated 24 years before, so this was probably David, the son; see Roger French, 'Sickness and the Soul', *The medical enlightenment of the eighteenth century*, (Cambridge, 1990), p. 100.

(12)   Thomas Glass was awarded his MD under Dr C. Oostendijk Schacht. See Leyden University archives, reference ASF 415, p.300.

(13)   Atrophy in general, Phthisis of the Lungs, and those Particular Diseases, which lead to it. See appendix.

(14)   William Munk, *Roll of the Royal College of Physicians*, p. 52. From his phraseology it is evident that Munk had copied Parr's words; as librarian of the Royal College of Physicians, Munk had ready access to Parr's MS.

(15)   *Ibid*.   P.J. and R.V. Wallis, *Eighteenth Century Medics*, (VadeMecum Press Ltd, 1988). Hereafter Wallis.

(16) R.Brookes, MD, *The General Practice of Physic*, (London, 1754), Vol.II,p.187.

(17) John Andrew, *The practice of inoculation impartially considered...*, (Exeter, 1765), p. 68.

(18) See C.W.Boase, *Bibliotheca cornubiensis* (1882), III, p. 1029. The dispute was essentially about the valuation of an estate owned by Pitfield which Andrew was proposing to buy. Pitfield was an apothecary, one of Thomas Glass's executors; William Chapple was Secretary to the hospital and was invited by Andrew to value the property. The argument became extremely heated and occasioned 'three pamphlets and twenty-four fugitive publications'.

(19) An Apothecary, *Observations on the state of the dispute between a physician and an apothecary* ... (London, 1765).

(20) See Kenneth Dewhurst, *Dr Thomas Sydenham* (1624-1689) (London, 1966), p.71.

(21) It was Parr himself that had suggested that the Latin of the *Commentaries* was that of a Mr Wood, a schoolmaster of Bampton, and not Thomas's own. Any 'malevolent suggestion' therefore came from him.

(22) William Munk, *Western Times*, (October 13, 1855), p.8.

(23) George Oliver, *The History of the City of Exeter*, (Exeter, 1861), pp 161-165.

(24) J. Delpratt Harris, *The Royal Devon and Exeter Hospital*, (Exeter, 1922) p.6.

(25) DRO Act Book of the Chamber XIV p.99. Quoted by permission of Exeter City Council.

(26) *Ibid* p.101

(27) DRO 1260F HM 8. Quoted by permission of Exeter City Council.

(28) Delpratt Harris *op. cit.*, note (24) p.7

(29) DRO Act Book XIV p.101 A. Quoted by permission of Exeter City Council.

(30) Munk, op. cit.. note (22). Parr *passim*. Wallis *passim*.

(31) Parr, *passim*.

(32) Delpratt Harris, op. cit., p.9. Wallis *passim*. Joseph Foster, *Alumni Oxoniensis*, (Oxford, 1891), passim.

(33) DRO Receivers Vouchers Box 516 1741-42. Quoted by permission of Exeter City Council.

(34) Parr, *passim*.

(35) DRO Act Book XIV p.190 A.. Quoted by permission of Exeter City Council.

CHAPTER II
Bedford House and its Social Circle
The perspective of Bartholomew Parr; jaundiced and less jaundiced

*Be thou as chaste as ice, as pure as snow,
thou shalt not escape calumny.*

HAMLET.

On arrival at Exeter, Thomas and Mary Glass took a lease on a part of Bedford House, a mansion built in 1532 by Lord Russell, later Earl of Bedford. It was built on three sides of a courtyard; a drive, flanked by trees, led from the gatehouse on the south side, through an archway under the central block, grandly embellished with the Bedford coat of arms, to the stables and gardens beyond. The house had historic, indeed royal, connections; in 1644 Charles sent his queen to Exeter, with its Royalist sympathies, for safety during her confinement; the baby princess was born at Bedford House on June 16 and baptised Henrietta Maria in the cathedral in July.

Part of one wing of the house was occupied by Benjamin Heath (1704-1766), the wealthy son of a wealthy fuller and merchant; born a Baptist, he waited until both parents had died until in 1729 he changed his allegiance to the Church of England. He was a classical scholar, lifelong bibliophile, and Town Clerk of Exeter from 1752 until his death. In 1730, at the age of 26, being left a fortune of £30,000, Benjamin set off on the Grand Tour, collecting a bride aged fourteen on the way, Rose Marie, the daughter of a Genevese merchant. He settled in Exeter but had no liking for business, preferring the less worldly atmosphere of books and, it is said, living the life of a valetudinarian. Perhaps his preoccupation with his health encouraged him to cultivate Thomas Glass as friend and even more as neighbour. Rose Marie had thirteen children in twenty years, and lived to the age of ninety. Of their seven sons, five survived, one becoming headmaster of Eton and one of Harrow; only three of their six daughters lived out their childhood.[1]

Another wing of the house was occupied by Bartholemew Parr, senior, (1713-1800), one of the surgeons who first formed the surgical staff of the Devon and Exeter Hospital, a former pupil of Smellie and a skilful accoucheur;[2] an additional bonus for Benjamin Heath in his choice of home.

Bartholemew Parr, junior, (1750-1810) was born at Bedford House to the surgeon's second wife. This family too were dissenters, the grandfather, also Bartholemew, having been a dissenting minister of Rewe and Clyst St George. As such, in 1809 the grandson was disqualified from election to the Exeter

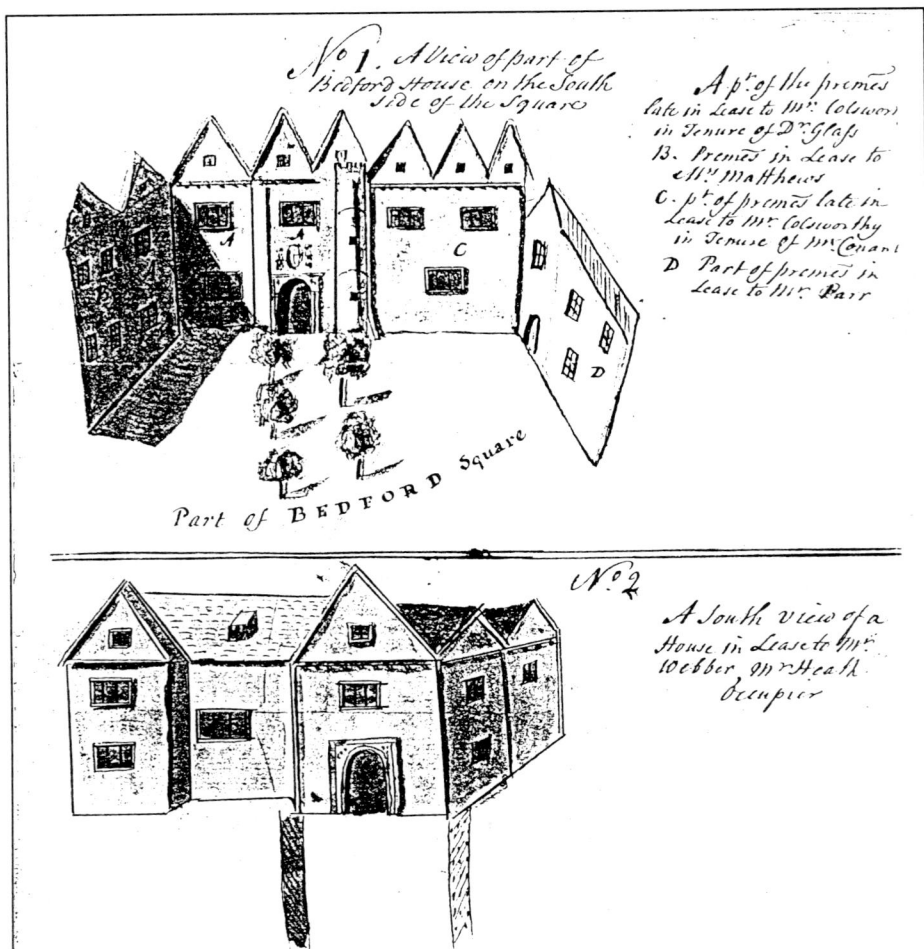

No 1. A View of part of Bedford House on the South Side of the Square

A pt. of the premises late in Lease to Mrs. Colsworthy in Tenure of Dr. Glass
B. Premises in Lease to Mr. Matthews
C. pt. of premises late in Lease to Mr. Colsworthy in Tenure of Mr. Conant
D Part of premises in Lease to Mr. Parr

Part of BEDFORD Square

No 2

A South view of a House in Lease to Mr. Webber Mr. Heath Occupier

Bedford House, Exeter. Mid 18th century (by kind permission of the Marquis of Tavistock and the Trustees of the Bedford Estate).

Chamber;[3] no doubt too, this determined that his medical training should take place in Edinburgh, where he graduated MD in 1773.

Bedford House was pulled down in the same year to make way for Bedford Circus. The Heaths had moved to Teignmouth in 1762, the Parrs, father and son, moved into Bedford Circus as it was completed, an architectural treasure, destroyed by enemy action in 1942. Thomas and Mary Glass moved to Bartholemew Yard, but retained a lease on the garden they had enjoyed at Bedford House.

Thomas Glass retired from his hospital appointment in 1775 and was succeeded by the young Parr; there seems to have been no very obvious explanation for Parr to bear a grudge against his professional senior and erst-

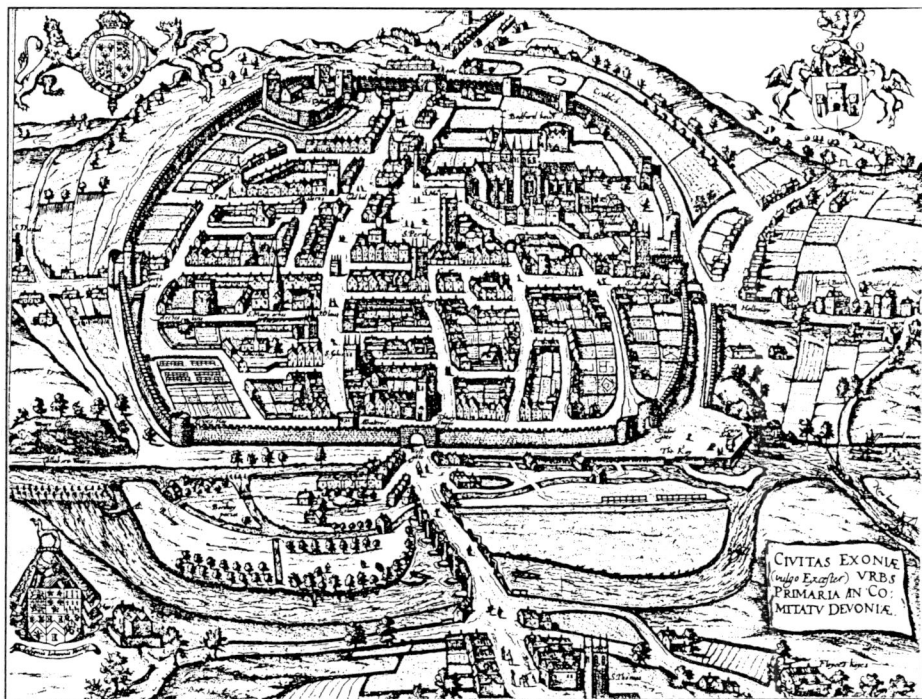

Exeter 1618. Bedford House to north of the cathedral
(by kind permission of Exeter Central Library).

while neighbour, so frequently to be revealed in his appraisal of Thomas Glass's life.[4] It is tempting to assume that there was resentment because no private practice was passed on at the time of the hospital succession, as he hints at in this passage, afterwards deleted from the manuscript version of his lecture:

> To me, who afterwards became a Candidate for Practice, Dr Glass resigned his Place in the Hospital, for which I owe him my Thanks; but they would have been more Cordial could I have perceived the favour to have been totally unsullied by personal motives and his own interest.

Other passages are nothing if not pejorative:

> His hand was always open, and the proffered fee was always ready; nor in the Excess of this fulness, did He always distinguish between the Friend to whose Interest he had been materially indebted, and whose pittance was scanty, between the industrious and less opulent Tradesman, and the Man of Rank, the Wealthy and the Independant.

He must have thought that this also was too strong to be handed down to posterity, for it also was deleted. This however was left intact:

33

As Dr Glass passed his Life in a Provincial Town, as his Talents were not splendid, and his Philosophical acquisitions were inconsiderable, his Fame could scarcely be expected to extend far beyond his own neighbourhood. Yet in 1776, when the Royal Society of Medicine was established in France, by the last unfortunate Louis, Dr Glass was chosen a Foreign Associate, an Honour bestowed indeed with some profusion, but not disgraced by an improper Choice. ...Yet this compliment, received with peculiar complacency, was followed by no literary Exertions; and no contribution to the Society followed. The Commentary on Celsus which had been for some time finished, was designed for this new Society, and to be printed at their Expence. I know not whether it was offered; but it certainly made no part of their Plan, and the offer, if made, must have been declined.[5]

And yet, as a younger man, living at close quarters with Glass, Parr must have had considerable respect, even admiration for his neighbour. In 1773 he chose a topic for his Edinburgh MD dissertation *de Balneo*, which followed Glass's interest in hot and cold bathing; furthermore he saluted in Latin 'That most illustrious man, Thomas Glass, most renowned of doctors', and added a fulsome dedication. Two years later he succeeded Glass at the hospital, in eleven years Glass was dead and in seventeen he proceeded to demolish his character, continuing with another passage, deleted in part:

His mind and body began at last to fail; but the World, little aware of their Mutual influence, ran eagerly to our worn out Veteran, who with equall eagerness met their added advances [caught the fee almost eluding his grasp. This indecent eagerness, this value passion continued to the last moment, was equally disgracefull to the Profession, and, often injurious to the Patient. But] [deleted].

Such were the Events of a Life little varied by extraordinary accidents, unadorned by splendid occurrences; of a Life externally prosperous but scarcely in any period of it happy. To toil for preeminence, for Fame and Affluence; to succeed in a degree which the most sanguine expectations could scarcely have suggested; and to taste of the cup only, when dashed with the poison of domestic misfortune, can scarcely be styled fortunate. Yet tho' this interchange of success and Disappointment may afford reflections to the Moralist, it must be the present object to trace the Events to their Cause, to learn from the Example before us, what to aim at attaining, and what to avoid.

Throughout this narrative, the disapproving shadow of Bartholemew Parr, is seldom missing from the background, the doppelgänger with the pointing finger:

From the Facts recorded, it will be obvious, that Dr Glass's success was rather owing to a series of Events peculiarly fortunate, than to his

34

BARTHOLOMÆUS PARR

VIRO ILLUSTRISSIMO

THOMÆ GLASS, M.D.

APUD ISCAM DANMONIORUM

MEDICO CELEBERRIMO,

S.

Cum in Medicina tot tamque meritos affequuutus sis Honores, cum de Balneis Veterum ipse tanta cum laude tractaveris; haud opus est ut exponam cur has Studiorum Primitias, TE AUSPICE, publicare lubet. Qualescunque sint, eas animi grati, TIBIQUE devinctissimi, tanquam pignus offerre volo, et tuo nomini inscribere.   *Vale.*

Dabam Edinburgi, prid. Id. Junii.

Parr's dedication of his M.D. dissertation.

Talents, Labour, and Assiduity. Prudence had little share in concerting or bringing them to their fortunate issue. His reserve was not impenetrable; his manners not conciliatory; and He was respected for his medical Talents, rather than admired for his general knowledge. He possessed the confidence rather than the affections of his fellow Citizens: He was more respectable than amiable. His mind was indeed always of the sterner mould; [?] harshly severe rather than mildly affectionate. Yet perhaps such was owing to manner: somewhat in his appearance seemed an opposition to kindness; and sometimes inattention was mistaken for Cruelty. 'I did not tell him', says Dr Glass, speaking to me of a Patient, 'I could not say his Eye was lost: it would have affected him too much.' He forgot that I was present at the interview, that I had witnessed his telling the distressing Truth with little reserve.

This gentleness of Heart, of which his Countenance was so unfaithfull a Herald was not irregularly or hastily displayed. I have opposed the general opinion, that He was a severe Father, and as a Master He was hard and indulgent. His Charities were private, but they were numerous. His benevolence was not blazoned in the face of the Day; but it was judiciously directed and properly proportioned. I have reason to believe that many as object in distress blessed him as their unknown benefactor.

In his youth He was esteemed handsome, and a Picture still, I believe at Hillersdon, is said to confirm the opinion[6]. In advanced Life, an unpleasing Character deformed features naturally good. His apparent sagacity was sometimes sullied by a sarcastic sneer; the Lines of deep thought and penetrating judgment were debased by [the appearance of a selfish Cunning] [deleted] a more unpleasing Expression [added]. In each decision, the Physiognomist would not greatly err. His mind was strong, but not enlarged; His judgment was sound, but his views were [selfishly] [deleted] contracted.

In a professional view, these Lights and Shades were equally conspicuous. His medical Erudition was not extensive. He had read with attention, the antient Medical Works, and was chiefly conversant, among the moderns, with those who trod in the footsteps of Galen.

Now follows a transparent attempt to appear evenhanded, though he was unable to resist the occasional waspish sally:

Yet the medical knowledge of his early work he had matured with Care, and from his discriminating Sagacity, could apply his collective stores with equall accuracy and readiness. His retentive memory, and his unruffled observation enabled him to meet every exigency, by resources well adapted [and skilfully to direct] [deleted] to regulate the operations of Nature, in Circumstances, the most alarming. The distinctions,

36

which Ignorance can not comprehend and Indolence will not examine, were to him obvious, and neglecting an apparent or a forced Similarity, He directed his reserves to the disease and not to a name. To these facilities, he owed his well founded reputation, his Fame and his Fortune. The various steps between the first impression and the action were by Habit and skill so rapidly connected, that his Decisions appeared to [be] [deleted] the inattentive observer [added] hasty and undistinguishing.

If surveyed more closely and followed in subjects less familiar, and with which He was not daily conversant, He will appear slow, less accurate, and indecisive, except after long deliberation. Even in his professional departments, this indecision would sometimes appear, and his determinations have occasionally been so long delayed, that the Event, either fatal or fortunate, has anticipated the Determination. In a mind, slow, deliberate and discriminating, Scepticism approaches, before Age has cooled the Ardor, and checked the activity of the mind. In Medicine, from the numerous difficulties, which must daily occur, its arrival will be accelerated: for to Balance each will lead sometimes to a fatal Delay. In the practice of Physic there is often only a choice in inconveniences: to meet the most important with spirit and decision requires equall judgment and energy of mind. It was an Exertion, to which Dr Glass for many years before his death was unequall.

In this Country, He greatly reformed the Practice of Medicine, tho' seldom by his own Discoveries. In fevers, Sydenham was his guide; and to the regular use of Laxatives, rather than any new systematic Plan, his Success was owing. By these Medicines He was chiefly enabled to check the progress of Miliary Eruptions, and to prevent the Disease, when attended to early. Yet, in the Employment of Laxatives, was He, in his later years timid and indecisive. In two bilious Epidemics, I saw his Patients recover slowly and imperfectly, from the too cautious use of Purgatives; [for, at last, He would only keep the bowels moderately loose] [deleted]

In other branches of Science, Dr Glass's acquisitions were very limited. With Botany as a Science, He was unacquainted; of Chemistry, He had very slight superficial knowledge; and, in Natural Philosophy, his attainments were scarcely more than the common Elementary Systems, at that time peculiarly defective, could afford. In general Literature, He possessed only a faint outline, which enabled him to join in conversation, if without applause, at least without disgrace.

The Indecision and Scepticism which appeared in his professional Studies, was still more conspicuous in his metaphysical and [literary][deleted] religious Enquiries ... Causes of this kind probably led Dr Glass to that miserable state of fluctuation, which distinguished the last months of his painfull existence. In this period, he seems to have doubted, Hesitated, and sometimes changed his opinions, and these doubts probably added to his anguish. I have reason to believe that some other scruples [?]added equally to disquiet him. His conduct, tho' probably honest had not been especially generous. [He had taken the last Guinea from the Hands of industrious Poverty][deleted] He had in more than one instance, unjustly appropriated the Labours, and discoveries of others to himself...

Parr, so long after Glass's death, may have felt himself on safe ground in thus attempting to destroy his reputation, for there seems little doubt, from his constant carping, that this is what he intended, indeed the lapse of two hundred years scarcely conceals either his smugness or the evident enjoyment of the task. Mary, Glass's wife, was dead, as were all his brothers; of his family, only his sister, Elizabeth, was still alive at Tiverton and two of his married daughters, Melina and Ann. Apart from enhancing his own reputation by invidious comparison, weakening the encomia already heaped on his prey, it is difficult to understand Parr's purpose, other than to indulge his spite on someone he despised and envied. His account is probably safe when dealing with specific happenings, especially when supported by the word of others, but his value judgments must be suspect. The amendments to his manuscript may be due to conscience or to anxiety about his image in the eyes of his peers.

Richard Polwhele, a prominent member of the Exeter Literary Society, was almost certainly in Parr's audience, but it seemed to have had little adverse effect on him, for in 1806 he wrote:

But the fame of that very eminent physician, Dr Thomas Glass seems to have eclipsed that of Dr Andrew. I have never met with Glass's treatise "De Febribus", or his essay "On the Attributes of the Deity", but have frequently heard them mentioned with approbation...[7]

There is little doubt that Parr was a complex and perhaps unlikeable man; but he was not solely a literary iconoclast. He was the author of a massive book, *The London Medical Dictionary*, and contributed a large number of critical reviews to the *Medical and Philosophical Commentaries* and *The Annals of Medicine*. He was a F.R.S. of both London and Edinburgh. The customary anodyne obituaries in the local press and the entry in the *Dictionary of National Biography* are interestingly offset by an entry in Farington's Diary:[8]

Dr Parr, an eminent Physician of Exeter, who died yesterday, became a subject of our conversation. He was a man who had much literary knowledge and considerable practice in His profession, but His disposition was avaricious; He gave way to much sensuality, even to low, impure connections; and in the indulgence of his appetite He sought for luxurious foods. He appeared to be sensible that His constitution was giving way before he died, but this did not lessen His desire for such

38

gratification. A week before His death He ordered a goose, which was considered strong diet for an invalid. His professional practice was supposed to bring Him about £1500 a year, but He derived a fortune from other sources and was judged to be possessed of £80,000 or £100,000. Such was the account given me; another lesson of inconsistency. A man of a grave profession; a scholar much devoted to literary pursuits; one who had liberal intercourse with society, and whose business it was to study the human constitution; yet with all these advantages and guards against imprudence, He was said to be selfish and narrow in His mind; an epicure in His living; and to risk His constitution to gratify His passions.

Bartholemew Parr married twice, his first wife, Maria (née Codrington), died in 1803, at the age of 34, having given him two sons, both of whom entered the church; the second wife deserted him after six weeks, though she continued to correspond affectionately with his sons. Perhaps she should be credited with commendable perspicacity. One may note in passing that Maria Parr was the daughter of John Codrington (1735-1801), surgeon apothecary, a member of the Exeter Medical Society which had presented Glass with the Opie portrait, and signatory to the accompanying testimonial. He was also one of three apothecaries appointed as trustees of Glass's will, surely an indication of mutual friendship and respect. He was a member of the 'Society of Gentlemen' and the subject of a sonnet by Downman. Did his father-in-law's close relationship with Glass exacerbate an already slowly festering resentment? Was it significant that so many but Parr attracted a Downman sonnet? Farington implies that Parr's personality was flawed, was it perhaps pathological?.

Glass was not the only physician that Parr put down; Dr William Williams, who had died in 1740, ten years before Parr was born, was referred to thus:

Dr Williams had been the Medical Oracle of the West; but his only claim to the Character seems to have been his Sagacity in the Prognostics. He knew when to promise recovery, and when to pronounce the decisive doom, and He took care to insinuate, that each was in his power, if applied to early, and attended to scrupulously. In other respects, violent, and overbearing, severe and unrelenting, He made everyone bend to his caprices and prejudices.

On the whole Parr seemed to reserve his barbs for Glass and members of his own profession; he could be reasonably objective about others, so it is appropriate here to mention some members of the circle of friends of Thomas Glass and Benjamin Heath who were to be seen from time to time in one or other of their houses, and to whom Parr refers.

Alderman Thomas Heath, Benjamin's brother, was undoubtedly one such, and Parr speaks favourably of him, perhaps because his son, Mr Justice Heath, an important figure in the Exeter of his day, was Parr's contemporary:

> *... was bred in the commercial Line; but his Education had been liberal, and his mind was always active. Of his literary talents, we have only a specimen in his translation of the Book of Job. Yet his contemporaries speak of him as a Scholar, and a Man of general knowledge. He seems to have been well acquainted with the Human mind, and capable of gaining the strongest ascendancy over those He wished to bend to his purpose; and some Letters written by him, which have by accident reached me, show that his Ideas were clear and distinct, his Language perspicuous and pointed with classical precision. He conducted with consummate skill, the business of the Chamber and secured by the members which his Interest placed in that body, a constant majority ...*

Thomas Heath was twice mayor of Exeter, in 1738 and 1749, but it seems that his business suffered at the expense of local politics and he died relatively poor. The mayor was required to entertain on a lavish scale; his official functions included eighteen 'Monday Dinners' and four 'Great Dinners'. National events such as military victories, and royal anniversaries, weddings and births required the mayor to turn out in a manner befitting the dignity of a virtual city state. Accompanied by constables, staff-bearers and sergeants-at-mace 'in gorgeous robes and Hats superb of lace' the mayor processed in solemn procession. Equally fine were the sword-bearer, the aldermen in their scarlet robes and, two-by-two, the councillors in black.[9] The mayor-alderman on the one hand and the town clerk on the other made a formidable pair. The latter made a great reputation for himself in his successful and vigorous opposition to the cider tax, so unpopular in the South West.

Thomas Glass and the Heath brothers made the nucleus of a group of friends who met at Bedford House for conversation and companionship. The others consisted largely of clerics, so that when the topic of local politics was exhausted, one may be sure they moved on to matters spiritual and philosophical. Oxford in 1762 conferred on Benjamin a Doctorate of Civil Law, thus finally expunging any taint of his dissenting origins.

Notable in this circle was The Reverend Zachariah Mudge, Prebendary of Exeter and Vicar of St. Andrew's in Plymouth, regarded with great respect and affection by Dr Johnson. In 1769 Johnson wrote a generous obituary of him in the London Chronicle:

> *...a man equally eminent for his virtues and abilities, and at once beloved as a companion and reverenced as a pastor. He had that general curiosity to which no kind of knowledge is indifferent or superfluous; and that general benevolence by which no order of men is hated or despised.*[10]

Zachariah was an intimate friend of Joshua Reynolds, whose father and grandfather he had known well, and who had introduced him to Johnson. One of his sons was Thomas Mudge (1717-1794), the celebrated watchmaker, inventor of the lever escapement; his fourth son was Dr John Mudge (1721-1793) FRS, a well-known physician at Plymouth, with whom Johnson and Reynolds stayed when they visited Devon in 1762.[11] Though wellregarded as a physician at Plymouth, John Mudge had not had any formal training as a physician, purchasing his MD degree from Aberdeen, when over sixty. He was FRS, but this was in connection with his knowledge of optics and astronomy.

Archdeacon Sleech often visited, a great supporter of the new hospital from the outset; it was he who preached the sermon on the first anniversary of its foundation, to be published and sold for two guineas. He was Archdeacon of Cornwall and, according to Parr, was esteemed as a man of learning and of extensive classical attainments. Along with William Chapple, the hospital secretary, and William Pittfield, an apothecary, he was involved in the litigation with Dr Andrew.

The Reverend William Hole was another Archdeacon, he was Prebendary of Exeter and Archdeacon of Barnstaple. He had been delegated to enquire into allegations of scandalous behaviour against John Wesley, laid by the landlady of The Feathers Inn at Mitchell, in Cornwall, and her maidservant; the charge had been made against Wesley that he had told Mrs Morgan, the innkeeper's wife, that she was damned because she didn't know whether she was saved; furthermore that when the apostles went abroad to preach the gospel they were 'without expense' and signified his intention of himself being entertained in the same manner; finally he 'had said things with a maid of hers which were very improper to have been spoken to a young girl especially by a clergyman'. Surely a delicate affair, which ended on a note of anticlimax when the accusation was retracted. In 1791 his obituary in the *Gentleman's Magazine* said of him:

> ...*His mild and friendly temper, communicative, curious and cheerful conversation, extensive learning and unaffected piety would long be remembered by all who knew him with delight and veneration.*

His son, the Rev. Richard Hole (1746-1803), a minor poet and subject of a Downman sonnet, was a member of the 'Society of Gentlemen'.[12] Of the others mentioned by Parr, in the social circle centred on Bedford House, were the Weston brothers, Samuel and Stephen, sons of the Bishop of Exeter, a Mr Duer, a merchant trading in the West Indies and member of the hospital committee, and John Bradford, who of all of these seems to have been personally acquainted with Bartholemew Parr:

> *He was the intimate friend of my best friends, to his countenance and conversation I was much indebted in my earliest days, and I can reckon the hours I spent with him among the most pleasing and improving of my life. ... One of his most particular friends was the late Sir Richard Bampfylde, and to Mr Bradford's judgment, conciliating advice and*

> *friendly interference, many disagreeable domestic altercations were avoided; and public malice, or affected good nature, had little room for comments on their matrimonial disputes.*
>
> *... To Dr Glass, Mr Bradford was an early and sincere friend. He never lost sight of his interest, and the confidence which Sir Richard Bampfylde reposed in his medical abilities were at first owing to the recommendations of Mr Bradford. Many similar and very important services Dr Glass obtained by his interest; and it is with regret I must add, that this is not the only instance, in which at a future and more prosperous era, Dr Glass spurned the ladder, which contributed to raise him.*

Benjamin Heath and Thomas Glass had much common ground. Apart from living as neighbours, both had been converts to the established church from a baptist background and both basked in an aura of bookishness. Preoccupation with matters spiritual was a feature of mid-Enlightenment Britain, and no doubt the ambience of the cathedral and the prevalence of clerics within their circle fostered this; suffice it to say that both at various times published religious essays. The first of these was in 1740 when Heath published 'An Essay towards a Demonstrative Proof of the Divine Existence, Verity and Attributes of God', dedicated to Dr William Oliver, the Bath physician. In 1762, following the award by Oxford of an honorary DCL., he felt it his duty to enter upon a Refutation of Mr Hume's philosophy, which in Heath's view 'overthrew all truth and knowledge, all Religion and Morality'.[13] Parr reported that:

> *A few years after Dr Heath's death, about the year 1770, an anonymous pamphlet entitled Meditations upon the Attributes of God, and the Nature of Man was published with such a particular Designation, as fixed the Author to have been of this City. An Air of Mystery has always surrounded it. Dr Glass, tho' He seldom scrupled to avail himself of the Labours of others, never claimed it; and when attributed to Dr Heath, He neither admitted nor denied the assertion. After much enquiry, as well as a strict attention to the external and internal evidence, I have as little hesitation in tracing the publication to Dr Glass. He had probably particular reasons to consider it as wholly in his own power.*

Parr considered this pamphlet a masterly defence of Necessitarianism and the public outcry that it occasioned to be wholly unjust, but he took an altogether different view of the work that followed in 1772, undoubtedly published by Glass, *A View of Revealed Religion as it stands to the Reason*. He pointed to the glaring difference in style and concluded that they came from different hands, notwithstanding that 'in the title it was attributed to the author of the former work'. True to form Parr roundly attacks the pamphlet, confirming flaws in Glass' character, with that most damning smear of all, hypocrisy:

> *... it might be recollected that Dr Glass, tho' bred a Dissenter, had turned with a suspicious rapidity to the Church, had for years frequented it, with peculiar zeal, joined with unusual fervour in all its offices, participated with a punctual attention its most Solemn Sacraments. This Avowal therefore, this defence of Arian, almost of Socinian, principles must convict him of an Hypocrisy as disgraceful as the avowal was imprudent.[14]*

There is one possible explanation for Parr's demolition of Glass's reputation that has not been discussed; that , paradoxically, it was due to a misguided sense of altruism. One of Parr's teachers at Edinburgh had been the celebrated and charismatic John Gregory, senior, (1724-1773), who at the age of forty was made Professor of Physic. In 1769 he delivered six lectures entitled 'Observations on the Duties and Offices of a Physician and on the Method of Prosecuting Enquiries in Philosophy.'[15] These were published anonymously, probably by one of his students, in 1770, and again in 1772, under his own name.

Particular attention has been drawn to this work by John Truman,[16] emphasizing Gregory's stature as an early pioneer of medical ethics, a torch passed on to his students, who included Thomas Percival of Manchester, and two who practised with distinction in America, Samuel Bard and Benjamin Rush.

Gregory, both philosopher and physician, and a flower of the Edinburgh Enlightenment, set out his guidelines with a compelling logic. He was certainly held in high regard by Parr, who qualified in the year that Gregory died. In the last paragraph of his MD dissertation he paid Gregory a touching compliment, mourning his loss.[17] Some of his precepts may well have continued to echo in his ears:

> *It is difficult and painful for men to give up favourite opinions, the children of their youth; to sink from a state of security and confidence into one of suspense and scepticism. Accordingly few physicians change either the principles or practice they first set out with.*
>
> *... We sometimes see a very remarkable difference between the behaviour of a physician at his first setting out in life, and afterwards when he is fully established in reputation and practice. When beginning the world he is affable, polite, humane and assiduously attentive to his patients; but when in process of time he has reaped the fruits of such behaviour and finds himself above the world and indepedent, he assumes a very different tone; he becomes haughty, rapacious, careless, and sometimes perfectly brutal in his manners.*

Gregory recommended 'an absolute contempt of the authority of all great names, in everything but matters of fact'. He stated:

> *... A bigotted attachment to certain great names in the learned world has done remarkable mischief to science.*

43

... Another obstacle to the improvement of science, similar to the former, has been a blind and superstitious veneration for antiquity.

... Boerhaave, Hoffmann, Stahl, and every systematic writer exclaim against theories, meaning one another's theories; for each of them explains, though in different and   opposite manners, the proximate cause of every disease they give account of, and the mode of operation of every remedy they prescribe, upon principles entirely hypothetical.[18]

These words fell upon Parr's ears when flushed with youthful idealism. May they have been the cause of a bitter disenchantment when he suddenly saw his former hero in a new light? A crusty old reactionary, who had denied him the goodwill of some of his private practice when he succeeded him at the hospital. A slavish disciple of Boerhaave, looking backwards still further to the increasingly suspect tenets of Galen and Hippocrates. Can paranoia not arise from the accretion of many thin layers on an insignificant nucleus, the resultant system being entirely logical to the subject? Is this the way it was with Parr?

After Glass's death, Parr himself presented or bequeathed many medical books to the cathedral library from his own collection. Among them are both editions of John Gregory's *Observations on the Duties and Offices... and his Elements of the Practice of Physic.*[18] There are also some interesting manuscript works, a *Course of Lectures on the Practice of Physic, Delivered in the University of Edinburgh in the winter of 1770-1771,* in three volumes. With these are two volumes of *Clinical reports of patients treated in the Royal Infirmary of Edinburgh by Doctors Gregory and Cullen.* These refer to 1771/72 (mainly Gregory) and 1772/73 (Cullen alone). Although, as Truman points out, lecture notes were often taken verbatim by professional scribes for sale to students, careful inspection of all these manuscripts shows a remarkable similarity in hand-writing to each other, and to Parr's own, suggesting that they may have been his own notes.[19]

Notes

(1)   *Dictionary of National Biography*: Benjamin Heath.

(2)   J. Delpratt Harris, *The Royal Devon and Exeter Hospital,*(Exeter, 1922), p. 85.

(3)   Robert Newton, *Eighteenth Century Exeter*, (Exeter, 1984), p.38.

(4)   Bartholemew Parr, *Biographical Anecdotes of the late Doctor Glass of Exeter*, 1795, Manuscript in library of Royal College of Physicians, London. Deletions and additions by Parr are indicated by square brackets.

(5)   The Celsus manuscripts are dealt with in chapter nine.

(6)   This portrait by Hudson is in the possession of Lord Borthwick, of Crookston, Midlothian, a descendant of Mary Glass, Thomas's eldest daughter. See chapter eight.

(7)   Richard Polwhele, *The History of Cornwall*, (London, 1806), p.128

(8)   *The Diary of Joseph Farington*, 1810, November 23rd, (London, 1926).

(9)   Robert Newton, *op. cit.*, p.46.

(10) James Boswell, *The Life of Samuel Johnson*, (London, 1901), Vol. 3, p.151.

(11) *Ibid*, Vol.1, p.250. And Stamford Raffles Flint, *Mudge Memoirs*,(Truro, 1883), p.80.

(12) *TDA* LXXXVIII, p.130.

(13) *DNB*, Benjamin Heath. See also Sir W.R. Drake, *Heathiana*, (London, 1881). Glass bequeathed his valuable collection of medical books, some three hundred and fifty in all, to the Exeter Cathedral library.

(14) The location of these of these two tracts is given in the Introduction, note 15. Arian refers to the doctrine of Arius of Alexandria, who denied the full divinity of Christ. Socinians deny the existence of the Trinity and also the divinity of Christ. Necessitarianism denies free will and maintains that all action is determined by antecedent causes.

(15) John Gregory, *Observations on the Duties and Offices of a Physician and on the Method of Prosecuting Enquiries in Philosophy*, (London, W.Strahan and T.Cadell, 1770).

(16) John T Truman, 'The compleat physician: John Gregory MD (1724-1773)', *Journal of Medical Biography*, 1995; 3; 63-70.

(17) Bartholemew Parr, *de Balneo*, MD dissertation, 13th June 1773. The passage relating to Gregory occurs in the last paragraph.

...Horum vero unum e medio sublatum adhuc lugemus! Virum summa humanitate, summa doctrina, insignem; GREGORIUM dico, quem hic commorasse sat erit; ecquid enimmeritis ejus nostrove respondeat moerori?

(...Truly we mourn one of these [his teachers] exalted above the common herd! Let me single out a man, full of humanity, full of learning; I speak of GREGORY, who will readily be called to mind; is there anything that can match either his merits or our grief?).

(18) Gregory, note (15) passim.

(19) Parr, note (4). A Xerox copy of his manuscript is in Exeter Cathedral library, providing an extended example of his handwriting.

CHAPTER III
Smallpox Inoculation

For out of olde feldes, as men seith,
Cometh al this newe corn fro yeer to yere;
And out of olde bokes in good feith,
Cometh al this newe Science that men lere.
GEOFFREY CHAUCER,
The Parlement of Foules.

Perhaps, along with the institution of the voluntary hospitals and the gradual elimination of magical and superstitious substances from the pharmocopeias, smallpox inoculation, that is the transfer of infected material from a person with the disease to one who had not had it, was the most significant development of the medical enlightenment of eighteenth-century Britain.

Smallpox, prior to the institution of inoculation and later vaccination, had been one of the major scourges of mankind; it had a high mortality, caused blindness and severe disfigurement. It was recognised, of course, that an attack of smallpox, however mild, conferred immunity from further attack; the main causes for concern and enquiry was whether inoculation was safe and whether it was more effective than the natural smallpox; in this respect it stimulated the collection of vital statistics, itself a beacon of medical progress. Leaving aside the ancient practice of inoculation in China, reports of its use in the Near East had filtered through to the Royal Society in London in the early years of the century, before Lady Mary Wortley Montagu lit the fuse by her celebrated letter in 1717.[1] For it was undoubtedly she that set in train the events that, gathering momentum, thundered down the century until they rolled snowball-like to the feet of Edward Jenner in 1796.

For some time it teetered on the brink of acceptability, the only people to benefit being young members of the royal family, young aristocrats and, para-doxically, six condemned criminals; by 1728 only 897 inoculations had been recorded in England and Scotland with 17 deaths.[2] It was Suffolk that provided the epicentre from which the practice spread, leaving in its wake a furore of ecclesiastical and medical outrage; here Robert Sutton(1707-1788) and his six sons developed the process with astonishing success and doubt-less considerable commercial reward. Even so it was 1757 before Robert Sutton seriously got underway with an advertisement in the *Ipswich Journal* of April that year; and prior to that scattered foci had been appearing in isolated areas of the country. Thomas Dimsdale(1712-1800), the celebrated inoculator of the Empress of Russia, said in 1767 that he had been inoculating regularly for 'upwards of 20 years'.[3] At Exeter, in 1765, Dr John Andrew in his *Practice*

46

of Inoculation[4] makes it clear that he had started this practice in 1741. This was the year of the foundation of the Devon and Exeter Hospital and it was one of the servants of Dr Alured Clarke, founder of the hospital, who was one of his early patients. Andrew stated that the prejudice against inoculation was so great that 'I was obliged to practise as it were in the Dark, visiting my Patients only by Night,' consequently he sought a written order in the Dean's own hand absolving him from possible blame

Winchester, Nov. 19, 1741.

Dear Sir

With regard to Margaret, I do here under my Hand, clear the Doctor and Apothecary of all intentional, or actual Guilt, of any Thing that may happen to her, in the Course of their lawful Employments.

When I left Exeter, she was very desirous of being inoculated. I hope nothing has happened that can intimidate her. A Doctor came here t'other Day, and produced a List of sixteen hundred Persons, who were inoculated between Farnham and Chichester, and the intermediate Country, of which I believe there were not six Miscarriages. In short, if you think her a proper Subject, and she is really willing to submit to the Operation I earnestly desire it; and doubt not of God's Blessing on so reasonable an Attempt. But it is with this sine qua non, that nobody, not even her Fellow servant, may know it is by Inoculation, till the Prejudice against it are a little more worn off.

Andrew goes on to say that Margaret was the Dean's cook, aged 41, very corpulent, and 'in Appearance, an improper Subject for Inoculation, however she went thro' the Distemper without any bad Symptom'.

He maintained that the inoculated smallpox seemed to be attended with less danger than the natural, because the infection was communicated by mild pus, through slight superficial incisions, to sound healthful bodies, properly disposed for its reception; also in the best season of the year, at a favourable time of life, and where a proper regimen could be observed during the days prior to the disorder.

It was his practice, whenever the person to be inoculated was of a full sanguine habit, to order blood to be drawn, to give three or four doses of purging physic with a few grains of calomel, at proper intervals, and an alterative medicine, with some preparation of antimony, every night, on the days that no purging physic was taken.

He admitted that the necessity for these measures was not universally accepted; Dr Wall of Worcester, for instance, told Andrew politely that he would hesitate to use mercury and antimony, and that there was no more than one case in ten that required any further preparation than some gentle evacuations and a little circumspection in regard to diet and regimen.

A letter from John Huxham, dated January 23, 1765, quoted in the tract, initially supports Andrew, since he says he seldom fails to give a mercurial purge or two, prior to the inoculation; and sometimes his antimoniated aethiops, especially when a verminous seminium, foul obstructed viscera, or glands were suspected. On the other hand, in the case of healthy young persons, he seldom gave more than a few gentle purgatives, enjoining them to a light easy diet, abstinence from flesh or fish, for a few days, and carefully guarding them against violent exercise and taking cold.

Andrew found that a mercurial purge, even to young persons, had the advantage of causing the evacuation of worms.

The preparation and management by individual inoculators, being both arbitrary and idiosyncratic, necessarily varied enormously. The Suttons paid attention to diet, but were very secretive about their medicines. A great deal of guesswork and surreptitious testing went on, but in the milieu of the day no one accused them of unethical practice; though when Daniel Sutton built a chapel for his patients in May 1766, and employed the Rev. Robert Houlton, at a salary of 200 guineas a year, to preach sermons in praise of the Suttonian System of Inoculation, no doubt some eyebrows were raised.

In May 1762 Sutton announced a new improved method of inoculation, a new and more effective secret medicine, and that his son, Robert junior, had joined him in practice; allied to this was the cold water treatment, disapproved of by Thomas Glass, and vigorous exercise in the open air.[5]

John Andrew gave precise details about dietary restrictions, before and after the operation, which he describes thus:

> *The Preparation being finished, the Operator must make an Incision in each Arm, with a Lancet, just deep enough to wound, but not to penetrate the Skin, about half an Inch long, into which is put a small Thread, impregnated with variolous Matter, and bound on pretty tight, during sixteen or eighteen Hours.*

And he gave a careful account of medication, bleeding where necessary, purging and clysters, in a meticulous programme, normally lasting about twenty-one days. He said further:

> *During the course of Twenty three Years, I have inoculated more than three hundred Persons, in the above Method, not one of whom has miscarried; and in my whole Practice I have only lost one, whose Case being frequently mentioned to the Prejudice of Inoculation, it may not be improper to give some account of it here.*
>
> *This Person was a promising Youth, of nine Years of Age. He had been prepared at his Father's House, about thirty Miles distant, in the usual Manner (except the omission of Calomel); and being brought to Exeter, the Operation was performed September 27th, 1751; from which Time till Oct. 3d, he remained very well. In the Evening of that Day, the Symptoms, which usually precede the Eruption of the SmallPox, came on with some Degree of Violence, and continued,*

without any Remission, till the 7th in the Morning, when he brought off two large Worms; after which a Gleam of Hope appeared, but this was of very short Duration, for the most alarming Symptoms soon returning with greater Violence, in the Evening of the same Day, he died. The perpetual Vomiting he was afflicted with (from Worms, as I suppose, in his Stomach) made it impossible to give the least Relief; and to them I attribute his Death, for the few Eruptions that appeared, seemed to promise a favourable Sort of SmallPox....

...Among all that I have inoculated, not more than ten have have had any considerable Number of Pustules, only three have had the confluent Sort, and even these three had scarce any secondary Fever.

There follows some discussion about the consideration of age and the optimum time of year, the statistical evidence in favour of inoculation and objections on moral or religious grounds. According to his calculations, there had been about 700 people inoculated in Exeter since 1741 and of these only two had died; the one he had already mentioned and one other who was not his patient. He concludes with a statement concerning inoculation issued by the College of Physicians in London, translated from the Latin:

The College having been informed, that false Reports concerning the Success of Inoculation in England have been published in Foreign Countries, think proper to declare their Sentiments in the following Manner, viz. that THE ARGUMENTS, WHICH IN THE BEGINNING WERE URGED AGAINST IT, HAD BEEN REFUTED BY EXPERIENCE: THAT IT IS NOW HELD IN GREATER ESTEEM BY THE ENGLISH THAN EVER: THAT THE PRACTICE OF IT INCREASES GREATLY AMONG THEM: AND THAT THE COLLEGE THINK IT TO BE HIGHLY SALUTARY TO THE HUMAN RACE.

There follows only the postscript, referred to in chapter one, in which Glass and Andrew collaborated.

Andrew states at one point that the total number of inoculations carried out in Exeter between 1741 and 1765 was in the region of 700 and he himself had supervised 300 of these; in his postscript he gives a revised figure of about a thousand that he and Glass had carried out, between them. One may guess, therefore, at the sort of numbers with which Thomas was dealing; fairly small compared with those of many inoculators.

Glass's reputation as the greatest English authority on inoculation after Sir William Watson[6], must have been founded on something more than numerical experience, and it was probably his considerable reputation as a physician, and his carefully argued *Letter... to Dr Baker on the means of procuring a distinct and favourable kind of smallpox*. It is no doubt significant that he stated there that he had not lost a patient in many hundreds that had been under his care.[7] This letter certainly made an impact, for it seemed that the celebrated Dr George Baker, Royal Physician, had thrown down the gauntlet by his open letter and Thomas had picked it up. It was reinforced soon after when Thomas, later the same year, followed up with *A second letter to Dr Baker on certain methods of treating the smallpox during the eruptive state*. Both letters disclose a wide-ranging familiarity with all the published work on the subject, providing a digest of received wisdom, together with some intelligence reports of information leaked from the Suttonian camp.

Such was the state of confusion about the rights and wrongs of smallpox inoculation, both medical and ethical, that a number of wellknown physicians had held back. Baker, later Sir George Baker and another Devonian, was one of these, and published in 1766 *An Inquiry into the Merits of a Method of Inoculating the SmallPox, which is now practised in several Counties of England*, a copy of which he sent to Glass. Baker was understandably puzzled by the fact that some operators instituted a rigorous dietary and medicinal regime of preparation and aftertreatment while others did little or nothing; and he was particularly concerned by:

> ... *receiving an account of the ill success, which has lately attended Inoculation at Blandford, it occurred to me, that some benefit might possibly accrue to Mankind if the Public had an opportunity of comparing the different result of different management.*
> ... *Out of 384 who were lately Inoculated at Blandford, 150 were poor people, for whom the parish paid the inoculator. Not one of these had the confluent SmallPox, not one died. Of the rest, a great number were in danger from the confluent SmallPox, and thirteen died.*

Dr Pulteney,[8] a local physician, had been questioned by Baker; he had not in fact carried out any of the inoculations and his opinion was set out in the form of a letter dated June 21, 1766. In this he pointed out that the smallpox had lately prevailed over many parts of the west of England and that at the time the smallpox broke out in Blandford there were at least 700 who had not had that disorder. When this happened in the first week of April there was universal hurry and precipitation and a rage for inoculation, a great demand despite contrary advice by local practioners; moreover a preparatory course was despised and hot substances were given during the eruptive fever and the sick were deprived of fresh and cool air. The implication was that the poor who had been paid for by the parish, thus presumably having minimal treatment, had paradoxically done very much better than those who had paid the inoculator.

Glass acknowledged with thanks the receipt of Dr Baker's *Inquiry* and took the opportunity of setting out his own views in the form of the two open letters, tracts in effect, respectively 72 and 55 pages long. He started by saying that he had himself been endeavouring to inform himself of the improvements (rather coyly, it seems) made by a certain Person and his sons, whose surprising success had engaged and well deserved the attention of the Faculty. He acknowledged that the discovery of this secret, which was said to have been successful in nine thousand instances, without a single miscarriage, would be of no small importance to the public; especially if the same should answer, as there is reason to hope it may, in the natural smallpox. In that he said he entirely agreed with Dr Baker as well as in 'our Endeavours to render our Art still more beneficial to Mankind'. His own inquiries into Suttonian methods appeared largely to confirm Baker's information; as with Andrew, diet, which could hardly be kept a secret, was described in considerable detail, the medication was secret and thus begged speculation. Glass was known to be greatly in favour of sweating medicines (sudorifics) in the event of fever occurring in the post-inoculation pre-eruptive phase; he was sure one of the secret medicines was in fact a sudorific and that this was perhaps the one factor that marked out the Suttonian system from that of other operators and the reason for its success:

> ... The Patients, who had a considerable degree of fever, and felt themselves much out of order, were permitted to lye in bed. An Apothecary of my acquaintance, who visited his Hospital last year, found three of them in bed with this condition: and he saw the Matron of the house give each of them a small tumbler of liquor, and was informed by her, they were to continue in bed until the eruption appeared.
>
> The liquor she gave them had the appearance of fair water, and tasted somewhat like Sherbet; they called it Punch. The inside of the Pewterpot, out of which she poured it, was stained black, probably with the Acid. This liquor was given three or four times a day to all who had any considerable degree of fever before the eruption: the use of it was to make them sweat. The Operator himself informed my Friend, that by giving this Medicine to a Lad, who had tumbled into a pond of water, a little before the turn of the SmallPox, putting him on a flannel shirt, and sending him to bed, he had sweated him plentifully for five or six hours, and thereby prevented him from receiving any hurt from the accident.

Glass then quotes various examples that had led him to conclude that the exhibition of sudorifics at the critical time, i.e. about the seventh day after inoculation, when signs of fever and malaise appeared, went far in insuring a successful outcome; in particular, reducing the number of pustules, especially of the face, which he regarded as a favourable sign. The objective must be to produce 'a favourable and distinct kind of Pox'; the extraordinary success of the process must depend on something other than careful preparation and fresh air, because he knew operators who paid no attention to either of these, with equally good results. He hastened to say that this did not apply to the putrid fever of ordinary smallpox; as a true follower of Sydenham,[9] fresh, cold air was vital in this case. In some parts of Dorset and Somerset, he said, it was usual to inoculate persons first, and prepare them afterwards, by bleeding, purging and a low diet; thus perhaps explaining the attitude of the inhabitants of Blandford. After all, the Levant Practitioners, so it was said, used no preparation at all, seldom losing a patient.

It seemed therefore that it could be questioned whether any benefit was to be gained from preparation other than preventing:

> *the inconveniency and mischief that may arise from worms, and foulness of the bowels and stomach; and from fullness of the vessels, and thickness of the blood, when the Patient is attacked by the fever.*

Moreover, he was convinced that a patient may be reduced too low by preparation, as a certain degree of fever was necessary, stimulating the circulation and concocting, separating and expelling the vitiated and infectious matter. When the eruption was slight it was almost always preceded by, and attended with, an universal kindly sweat. In one person only, a servant maid in the late Dr Heath's family, he had observed the complaints and feverish heat that usually follow inoculation, to have been carried off by a profuse sweat lasting the most part of the succeeding night, without the appearance of a single pustule; yet she subsequently attended several people with the smallpox without taking the infection.

In Glass's view, far from the Suttons' recommendations of fresh air and cold water, in those with languid constitutions it was sometimes necessary to provide stimulation with cordial medicines; the indications being continual vomiting, giddiness, lowness of spirits, faintness, a weak pulse and little or no feverish heat. This observation would perhaps meet with the approval of a modern physician, who would hold that fever is a sign that the body is actively combating infection; contemporary eighteenth century wisdom required that fever was to be eradicated at all costs. He mentions a thirty-year-old lady, reduced low by preparation, exhibiting these signs and causing, it seems, a good deal of anxiety; she did not respond at first to cordial medicines, so their dose was increased; the next day she was given:

> *Cordial Confection, Theriaca, Contrayerva-root, volatile salts, strong Negus, hot Wine, given in no inconsiderable quantity, and Blisters applied to her back and arms. Not having the desired effect, her feet and ancles were wrapt up in Sinapisms,*[10] *the Wine was changed for French Brandy; of this, mixt with warm water, and by itself, she drank near three pints, before she had fever enough to compleat the eruption.*

The description of these somewhat heroic measures is interesting in that it is one of the few instances of an actual Glass prescription. Theriac was already coming under scrutiny, following William Heberden's reasoned and outright condemnation of it in 1745, but, old habits dying hard, it doubtless took a long time to gain general acceptance; the Edinburgh pharmocopeia omitted theriac in 1756, but it continued to appear in the London pharmocopeia until 1788.[11]

The essential art was to control the situation, neither allowing the fever to rise to high or to be ineffectually low:

How absurd, then, and pernicious is it for nurses to ply the sick with Sack and medicines, when their fever is very high and they are already suffocated with internal heat? And is it less absurd, or pernicious, for regular Practioners of Physic to treat their Patients with the cooling Regimen, and allow them nothing warmer than Crab's Claws, and Nitre, with a few grains, it may be of Contrayerva powder when their Pox are pale ... And when at the same time their pulse is weaker, and, it may be, slower, and their flesh less warm than in health?

...it is equally certain that many Patients, treated with the cooling Regimen, and given over, as past all Hopes of Recovery, by those under whose care they were, have been to the no small Disgrace of the Faculty, brought to life again by drinking Wine, strong Beer, or Brandy, which was given them by some old Woman contrary to orders, until their heart was well cheared, their blood warmed, and they fell fast asleep. So many instances of this kind have happened every where, and are so well known, that these are sufficient to account for the favourable opinion, the bulk of mankind entertain of Nurses' skill in managing the Small-Pox.

This would seem to have been an honest, open and perhaps courageous view to take.

He pointedly excluded from this policy the putrid malignant fever found in Jails and crowded Hospitals, the typhus of modern times. Here he referred back to his *Commentaries on Fevers*, in which he said this was better treated with purging medicines than with sweating. Digressing slightly on the treatment of typhus, he mentions an observation of Dr Brocklesby, in which he said that of a great number of sick soldiers, those housed in cold draughty shelters recovered much more rapidly than those housed in warm, draught-free, and more comfortable houses. Had he known that typhus is transmitted by the body louse, thriving in warm, overcrowded conditions a rationale would have been accorded to the observation.

It is pointed out that it is very rare for inoculated persons to develop the confluent type of smallpox, and when it occurs Glass thought it was due to the inoculator coming direct from visiting a patient in the acute suppuratory state; something that Glass took particular care to avoid, offering this as a possible reason for not having lost any cases in his own practice. Experience had taught him that:

Mercurial powders, and gentle purges, with a strict regimen, free use of air, and moderate exercise, are very little to be depended upon for preventing a bad sort of Pox when the infection is taken in the natural way.

Such statements indicate that though seemingly ambivalent in places there was nonetheless an underlying realism, even scepticism, with which he viewed conventional treatment, a pragmatist at all times.

53

Careful consideration of a number of methods, in particular the Suttonian, led him to conclude that the undenied success of the latter was due to:

> ... *its efficacy in preventing a numerous eruption, And that this event depends principally on the Patients being kept properly sweating in the eruptive fever by some medicines, which are administered for this purpose.*

There was discussion of the relative merits of various sudorifics and finally he commended the gentle sweating to be produced by the use of an external steam bath, particularly the 'elegant contrivance' of Mr Symons, a surgeon of Bath, which can be applied to the whole body up to the chin, without the patient being taken out of bed or obliging him to breathe hot moist air.

In the *Second letter to Dr Baker* Glass recapitulates his appraisal of Sutton's method, throwing in some mention of the methods of Drs Hancock and Dimsdale, in both of which cold water by mouth figures largely, the effect of which again is to procure a sweat, and here he quoted de Gorter.[12]

He pointed to the dangers of the 'new' method, which attached no importance to the appearance of any eruption, only to a slight swelling or inflammation of the punctured part; consequently in a number of cases (and he quotes the cases of two aristocratic ladies, the late Lady Morrice, and the Duchess of Boufflers), where both contracted smallpox within two or three years of the new method of inoculation, fatally in the former case.

There is further criticism of the exposure of patients to all weathers at every stage; since such patients are susceptible to other serious infections, particularly those arising from sore throat - 'the effects of the new method carried too far'. There were those who were prevented from making a proper use of their senses and reason by an over-fondness for what is new and very extraordinary, a medical failing repeated many times since then, part of humankind's innate love of paradox. It could be said that the whole business of inoculation was itself a paradox, the deliberate transfer of a distemper to a well person.

An inoculator who encourages his patients in every stage of the distemper, to walk about the streets and lead a normal life, may alarm the other inhabitants to the danger of infection and thus prompt them to themselves seek inoculation, to his considerable advantage. Here ethical shortcoming is implied, if not actually stated.

The views of Thomas Glass were well known to his contemporaries, Giles Watts for example in 1767[13] wrote:

> *It is the opinion of Doctor Glass, that the circumstance of Mr. Sutton's patients having the smallpox so extremely lightly, is owing principally to the administration of sudorifick medicines during the eruptive fever.*

I have a very high opinion of the abilities of Dr Glass, in matters of medicine in general, but I must beg leave to differ from him here. The medicines used by Mr. Sutton during the eruptive symptoms in inoculation seem to be no other (except purgatives) than Clutton's febrifuge spirit or tincture added to water in a certain proportion. And it must be confessed, that this medicine, especially if it be given warm, seems well calculated to excite sweat. This composition I have used with the utmost success, during the sickening of patients under inoculation. But then, on the other hand, I have many times observed, that those patients, who have not taken a single drop of this medicine, but have drank only weak tea, or lemonade, or some other cooling diluent liquor, have been equally inclinable to sweat as the others, and have had just as favourable an eruption too, as they have.

With all the wild rhetoric of a Welshman in any age, Evan David Llywythlan lambasted Watts in 1768, challenging every statement.[14] Of Glass he says:

I am glad you gave Dr Glass a wipe about his sudorifics during the eruptive fever; yet he will accuse you of doing the same thing by a quack medicine:
... Who was the real author of the Febrifuge Spirit or Tincture, I will not say; but, given with a certain proportion of warm water, you say, it seems well calculated to excite sweat. I hope Dr Glass will not see your book, or he will certainly recriminate. Hey day!

The previous year a curious anonymous document had appeared, *The Tryal of Mr. Daniel Sutton for the High Crime of Preserving the Lives of His Majesty's liege Subjects by means of Inoculation*. This was an unconvincing account of an imaginary trial at the College of Physicians, in which many of the principal characters in the smallpox saga were introduced as witnesses; among these were Baker, Ruston, Glass, Gatti and Daniel Sutton's personal clergyman, Robert Houlton, who had the leading part. There seems little doubt that it was all a rather clumsy publicity exercise, promoting the Suttonian method. Daniel Sutton evidently did not consider Glass' views incompatible with his own, and the words he puts into his mouth are a fair summary of his own views.

In the last three decades of the eighteenth century, that is until Jenner published his work on vaccination in 1798, inoculation became less and less controversial, the overall benefit having been demonstrated, backed up by the statistical studies of Jurin and Haygarth.[15] The City Chamber at Exeter was evidently convinced, for in October 1777 it:

Resolved unanimously that this Body will subscribe annually the sum of Ten Guineas towards Establishing and Maintaining a Hospital for Inoculating Poor Persons within this City.[16]

It did not become popular to the same extent on the continent; the only

English papers to be translated into German were those of Watson and Glass, in 1769.[17]

There is no doubt of the enthusiasm that was raised towards the latter end of the eighteenth century in the matter of smallpox inoculation; at last there was a medical intervention that seemed to work against this dreadful disease. Perhaps amongst the last personal communications that Thomas had on the topic was a long tract from Nicholas May, a Plymouth surgeon, in the form of a *Letter to Dr Glass*, extending to 199 pages.[18] May asked some pertinent questions, firstly whether the *Suttonian* medicines, if effective in inoculated smallpox, were equally effective in severe natural smallpox. Had any trials been carried out? He feared not: 'If they are found to be of truly antivariolous efficacy, why is their use so confined?'.

He asked in addition whether the success of the Sutton method might not depend in part on the very small amount of variolous matter used, no incision being made, the cuticle simply being raised with the tip of the lancet, one arm only being used:

> *In the old way of inoculating, the infectious matter was usually taken up by dipping a small dossil of cotton into the matter of several ripe pustules of a person in the SmallPox, or by running a large common needle, pretty well armed with thread through several ripe pustules, so as to make it sufficiently wet; from which cutting off small portions, in general about the size of a barleycorn, they inserted one such into each arm of the patient, by a slight wound made in the skin...*

Daniel Sutton had paid Plymouth a visit the previous summer for the purpose of inoculation and May had had an opportunity of seeing the effects of treatment at first hand, concluding that the secret medicines contained mercury and antimony. The first producing sore mouth, offensive breath, and salivation and the second a constant tendency to puke. Thomas's preferred sudorific was in fact a solution of tartar emetic[19], which in strong dosage produced catharsis and vomiting and in weak doses a gentle sweat.

Following on the first question he had posed, May had decided to use this to treat the natural smallpox:

> *Some time after the publication of your first Letter, addressed to Dr Baker, I was induced to make some experiments on the utility of the solution of Emetic Tartar, recommended by you near the conclusion; the effects of some of these experiments were as follow.*

A number of case histories follow, all but one being followed by recovery:

> *I am persuaded that we cannot have a more elegant and efficacious preparation.*

Notes

(1)   Lady Mary Wortley Montagu had seen inoculation carried out in Constantinople by local practitioners; the letter was written in 1717 to Mrs Chiswell.   She later persuaded Charles Maitland to inoculate her three year old daughter in 1721.

(2)   See David Van Zwanenberg, The Suttons and the business of inoculation, *Medical History*, 1978, 22, p.72.

(3)   Thomas Dimsdale, *On the present method of inoculation for the smallpox*. (London, 1767).

(4)   John Andrew, *The Practice of Inoculation impartially considered; its signal advantages fully proved* ... In a Letter to Sir Edward Wilmot, Bart, (Exeter, 1765).

(5)   Zwanenberg, op. cit., p. 76.

(6)   *Dictionary of National Biography*. Thomas Glass.

(7)   *A letter... to Dr Baker on the means of procuring a distinct and favourable kind of smallpox*, etc.,(London,1767), p.54.

(8)   Richard Pulteney MD, FRS (1730-1801). A distinguished botanist and physician of Blandford.

(9)   For Thomas Sydenham's cooling regimen in smallpox see Kenneth Dewhurst, *Dr Thomas Sydenham*,(London, 1966), p.104.

(10) A sinapism is a mustard poultice, generally applied to the calves of the legs or soles of the feet as a stimulant.

(11) Gilbert Watson, *Theriac and Mithridatium*, (London, 1956), pp. 142-147.

(12) Glass' reference is to de Gorter, *De Perspirat.*, Cap XI, 38.

(13) Giles Watts, *A Vindication of the New Method of Inoculating the SmallPox*,(London, 1767).

(14) Evan David Llywythlan, *Natural Observations on a Wonderful Pamphlet*, (London, 1768), pp. 19,20.

(15) For a recent account and commentary on inoculation of smallpox see Adrian Wilson, The politics of medical improvement in early Hanoverian London, *The medical enlightenment of the eighteenth century*, (Cambridge, 1990), p. 24.

(16) Devon Record Office, Exeter City Archives, Act Books, 21.10.1777.

(17) *Dictionary of National Biography*, Thomas Glass.

(18) Nicholas May, Junior, *Impartial Remarks on the Suttonian Method of Inoculation, in a letter to Dr Glass*, (London, 1770).

(19) Tartar emetic is also known as antimony potassium tartrate.

CHAPTER IV
Twelve Commentaries on Fevers

Explaining the Method of curing these Disorders,
upon the Principles of Hippocrates.

*Commentarii duodecim de febribus ad Hippocratis
disciplinam accommodati*

> *I set about reducing the Matter Hippocrates has left us, under such
> Heads as seemed to me most convenient, one of which was of Fevers.
> On perusing what I had collected together, I imagined that the History
> and Cure of Fevers, taken from Hippocrates, would be no unacceptable
> present to young Practitioners: For this Distemper is the most
> common, and the most fatal of all that afflict Mankind; and though
> some Physicians may have differed from Hippocrates as to the method
> of Cure, yet all allow that he was the best acquainted with the Signs of
> Diseases, and their Portent:*

Thomas thus sets his objectives in the preface to his major literary work, which was undoubtedly accorded much acclaim both during and after his life. First published in London in Latin in 1742, it was reprinted five times in the period up to 1788, in Amsterdam, Leyden, Jena and Leipzig, London and Paris, and Lausanne. It was translated into English by Nicholas Peters and published in this form in 1752; and a heavily annotated French translation, in two volumes, appeared in Paris in 1831, 89 years after its debut.

William Munk, compiler of *The Roll of the Royal College of Physicians*, and its librarian, possessed a Latin edition of the Commentaries formerly owned by Dr William Carter, Fellow of Oriel College, Oxford, and an 'eminent physician of Canterbury' in the eighteenth century. It had been freely annotated with comments in Latin, perhaps the most telling of which translates as:

> *Truly these commentaries are of the utmost use; at one time they were
> a reason for friendship between the author and myself. He learned the
> first elements of medicine at the feet of Boerhaave, and he is a man who
> is especially skilled in his same art.*

Munk, in 1855, wrote too, that at the time the Commentaries were published:

> *there were few medical publications, and to attempt to claim the atten-
> tion of the public was regarded as an attempt equally arduous and
> dangerous. Dr Glass's work however, was received with the highest
> applause, it proved him a man of extensive medical research, a patient*

*and accurate observer and a cautious reasoner. The Commentaries at
once established his credit and gave him the reputation of a scholar.*[1]

In these days it may seem hard to accept that in rather more than a quarter of
sufferers from lobar pneumonia in the nineteen thirties[2] the outcome was fatal,
so much more were fevers fraught with danger in the poverty-stricken and
highly insanitary conditions of the eighteenth century, presenting the physician with his greatest problems. Smallpox, typhoid, typhus, tuberculosis,
malignant sore throat stalked the streets, reaping a terrible harvest.

Although many medical worthies, including the incomparable Sydenham[3]
and Richard Mead[4] had written on fevers, the *Twelve Commentaries* were by far
the most comprehensive work on the subject at the time, extending to 280
pages or about 47,000 words. Of previously published books in England, it
was probably nearest in style to the *Nine Commentaries upon Fevers* of John
Friend, published in 1717.

It was not that the book was an epitome of catholic opinion on the causation and management of fevers. Glass eschewed contemporary
speculation, including that of Hoffmann[5] and Stahl,[6] although the former rates
a passing nod; he adopted the safer and more solid stance of the traditionalist, beating the Hippocratic drum as had Sydenham before him. Even the
great Boerhaave, his hero and mentor, is only briefly allowed his idiosyncratic
proposition of 'lentor', though he is quoted at length in the preface for his
avowal of 'that Fountain from which flows the Art of Presaging, and from this
the true Art of healing'. Hippocrates is referred to more than 50 times and
Galen is very frequently quoted; Friend, Mead and Huxham are all acknowledged, though the last was in connection with his essay on the Devonshire
colic, published in 1739[7] his *Essay on Fevers* was not to be published until 1750.

Huxham, at Plymouth, was of course a near neighbour. He too had been a
pupil of Boerhaave (though he graduated at Rheims) and took very much a
Hippocratic view of medicine. In the preface to his *Essay on Fevers* he doffs
his cap to Thomas Glass:

> *However it must be acknowledged, that all sober, regular, judicious
> Practice hath always been consonant to the Hippocratic Doctrine: as
> hath been shewn at large by the learned Dr Barker in his late Essay, to
> which I refer the Reader, and to Dr Glass's ingenious Commentaries for
> a Scheme of the Practice of Hippocrates.*

John Barker (1708-1749) had written an account of the recent (1741) epidemic
of gaol fever (typhus) in the west of England, which, it was said had spread
originally from prisoners at Exeter.[8]

Devotee of the Hippocratic Corpus as he was, Glass takes an eclectic view,
recognizing that the Divine Old Man was not one but many and that consequently the writings are full of inconsistencies and apparent contradictions,[9]
conveying both humanity and charm.

59

The Mechanism of Fever

It was part of Hippocratic doctrine that fever was an effort of nature to expel something hurtful from the body, either ingenerated or introduced from without.[10] This resulted in a violent commotion or perturbation in the system, followed by an evacuation from the skin and kidneys, with which the paroxysm ended. The commotion was ascribed to a fermentation, concoction, or ebullition, by which the noxious matter was separated from the sound humours. This resulted in a despumation or formation of a morbid scum which was then evacuated in various forms, in the sputum, via the bowel, in the urine, by haemorrhage, by sweating and so on.

Galen perpetuated these ideas and they had changed little by the dawn of the eighteenth century; they provided a plausible and ingenious model, if over-simplistic, which explained several of the phenomena of febrile eruptive illnesses. This was particularly so where one can postulate a peccant matter, producing general perturbation, multiplying itself as a ferment and at length thrown off at the surface by a direct depuration of the system. It fails however to explain febrile illness which is not productive of any skin eruption or indeed any evacuation of concocted material.

Boerhaave was aware of this difficulty and produced his own modification of the theory. Misinterpreting new discoveries in physiology, particularly the microscopical researches of Leeuwenhoek (1632-1723), he conceived that almost all diseases may be resolved into an introduction of any given parti-cles (or globules) of blood into a series of vessels into which they did not properly belong, a process he called *error loci*. The effect was that the sanguineous principles were broken down and rendered either too thin and serous or too gross and viscid. The viscidity of the blood he distinguished by the name 'lentor' and to the prevalence of this quality he ascribed the exis-tence of fever.[11]

Saul Jarcho[12] points out that at the beginning of Huxham's *Essay on Fevers* he reveals the difficulties of our eighteenth century predecessors in understand-ing fever. Thus he states that violent exercise will produce the febrile state; exposure to cold moist air will suppress perspiration, increasing the quantity of the humours, and a feverish habit [condition] will ensue. A large ingestion of wine or spirits will increase the quantity of the humours and will augment movement of the blood; this will produce fever such as is known to occur after a drunken debauch.

William Cullen (1712-1790) of Edinburgh listed the following as causes of fever-miasmata, contagion, heat, cold, venery, fear, dirt, putrefaction and bad air.[13]

Theories of the mechanism of fevers abounded in the eighteenth century; as more and more observations were made, so they were twisted and squeezed into uncomfortable shapes, as the feet of the ugly sisters were crammed into Cinderella's delicate slipper.

William Bynum[14] points out that there was a noticeable shift in the view of fevers between Huxham in 1750 and Cullen in 1770; the earlier emphasis being on treatment by depletion (thus reducing inflammation), and the latter by stimulation.

Commentary I
Of Fevers and their Difference

This is the shortest of all the commentaries and is the nearest the author gets to a nosology of fevers, based as was usual at that time on the periodicity of the febrile paroxysms, that is they were either Intermittents or Continuals. Fevers were also to be distinguished according to their causes, for example *Fever from Repletion* or *Fever from the Bile*, or from some remarkable symptom, as an *ardent Fever* or *Fever with Hiccup*. True to his theme:

> ... the great Parent of Physick was very little sollicitous about Names, and blames the Cnidian Physicians for being so particular about them: What he chiefly regarded was the Violence of the Fever, the Strength of the Patient, and the Tendency of the morbid Matter.

Thomas Glass's book, it should be said, lacks the richness of clinical observation of Huxham, or later, Cullen. He approached the subject from the 'right hand side' as it were, that is from the point of view of treatment, after the first four introductory commentaries. Refinements of treatment varied according to clinical circumstances.

Commentary II
Of Concoction and Crudity; with other Signs,
as well of Recovery as of Death.

This concept is essential to an understanding of eighteenth century ideas on pathology[15] and presents some difficulties to the modern ear:

> In every Fever great Regard is to be had to what Physicians call the Stages, or periods of the Disease, and these are four, viz: the Beginning, the Increase, the State, and the Declension ... Meat and Drink, then, received into the Stomach, continue in a crude state, until they are attenuated, dissolved, and digested; when they have undergone this Change, Concoction is finished in the first Passages. But the milky Humour thence prepared, which is there perfectly concocted, being afterwards carried into the Blood, is very unlike the Humour which flows in the Blood Vessels, and therefore is in this other Elaboratory of Nature, accounted crude, but when it has been farther prepared in the Vessels, and is changed into Blood, then it is no longer crude, but mature or concocted.

> *... In perfect Health it is certain,that both what is discharged from the Body, and what is retained within, are thoroughly concocted; and in Sickness, the nearer they are like what they were in Health, the nearer they are to a good concoction. Crudity is judged of from the Contraries. When there is any remarkable Crudity, the Body is some way or other disordered by it , and the greater the Crudity, the greater will be the Disorder. In Fevers, however, the Signs of Concoction and Crudity, are chiefly taken from the Stools, and from what is spit up, and from the Urine, but mostly from the latter.*

Several pages follow on the various signs of crudity in urine, care being taken to point out exceptional situations, strategically perhaps to cover the physician should nature take an unexpected course. So also are the stools described and likewise the sputa, and this is followed by a review of good and bad prognostic signs as set out in the Hippocratic writings.

Commentary III
Of the Crisis, and the Signs of its Approach

The Antients and their eighteenth century descendants were preoccupied almost to the point of obsession with the chronological minutiae of the feverish illness and this all hinged round the phenomenon of the Crisis:

> *In acute Diseases there frequently happens a sudden Change, either for Recovery or Death: This Change is generally preceded by a violent Perturbation, and some form or other of the following Symptoms. Very violent Pains of the Head, great Giddiness, a Delirium, deep Sleep, Noise in the Ears, Deafness, redness of the Eyes, Mists before the Sight, a false Perception of Flashes and Sparkles of Light, involuntary Tears, shaking of the lower Lip, a universal Tremor, a sudden Difficulty of Breathing ...*

It certainly had been held since antiquity that the crisis occurred on certain days rather than others, uneven days, for example, and the seventh in particular, a belief which lasted into the first four decades of the twentieth century.[16]

> *It having been observed that a Crisis happens more frequently, and that its Signs are more certain on some particular Days, the Antients have called these Days critical, among which the Septenaries were esteemed the most efficacious, and next the Quaternaries. The Septenaries are the seventh, fourteenth, and twentieth, for the second Septenary begins with the eighth Day, and the third with the fourteenth; ... But of all the critical Days, Galen thought the seventh the most powerful, next to that the fourteenth, ... The sixth has the worst Character of all, for the Crisis which happens on that Day is fatal, or at least extremely dangerous.*

Malaria was endemic in Britain at that time, notably in the fen country and the marshy areas around London; the characteristic tertian and quartan fever patterns would have accounted for many Intermittents unfamiliar today. Apart from that there would seem to have been a ritualistic or magical significance in these numbers; Glass hints at this and then dismisses it:

> But Celsus imagines that in this Affair the Antients laid a Stress on the Pythagorick Numbers, which were then in great Repute: However we find that regular Tertians by a constant Law, have their Fits on the alternate Days ...[17]

Commentary IV
Of Critical Evacuations and Abscesses

Almost all acute feverish illnesses produced an evacuation of noxious substances at some stage, as an expectoration, vomit, discharge of pus, sweating or diarrhoea. This often coincided with the crisis or at least with a paroxysm of fever. Artificial induction of one or more of these formed the basis of therapeutic intervention, so emetics; bloodletting, sweating and purgation became the prime measures to be taken, anticipating nature. The timing was all-important:

> Acute Diseases, when left to themselves, scarce ever end well without some remarkable Evacuations, or large Sediment in kindly Urine, or some critical Abscess. Such Disorders, according to Hippocrates, are carried off on a critical Day, by a Flux of Blood, by a plentiful Sweat, by a large Discharge of good coloured Urine, with a kindly Sediment, by loose mucous and bilious Stools, which are sometimes tinged with Blood; also by Vomiting and proper Abscesses. But Inflammations of the Lungs and Pleura, are chiefly removed by a free Expectoration of well concocted Matter; and when the same Disorder hath seized the Fauces, or the Glands seated near the Ears, such kind of Spitting is of the greatest Service.
>
> As to the particular Crisis which is about to happen, this may generally be foretold from the Season of the Year, the Epidemical Constitution, the Temperament of the Patient, and the Kind of the Disease, but chiefly from the Efforts of Nature, and the Tendency of the Humours. In general the more acute Fevers are usually terminated by Evacuations, and the more lasting by Abscesses.
>
> ... But Vomiting more frequently happens to Persons of a middle Age, and of a bilious Constitution, at the End of a hot Summer, and at the beginning of Autumn, when the Fever both begins with shivering and trembling, and has its Paroxysms like a Tertian Ague.
>
> ... the Disease was critically carried off by all these Evacuations...either

by a plentiful bleeding at the Nose, or by a large Discharge of Urine, with a copious laudable Sediment, or by loose bilious stools happening seasonably , or by a dysentery.

... Thus violent Pains in the Head, Giddiness, burning Heat, and such like Symptoms, are frequently carried off by a plentiful bleeding at the Nose in the Beginning of the Disorder.

... All those Evacuations which are improper for the Patient or the Disorder, and which do not at all alleviate the Symptoms, are to be reckoned among the Signs of a dangerous Distemper; if they add to them it is much worse, but worst of all, and most fatal, when the Matter discharged is much vitiated, and especially if it succeeds some pernicious Symptoms about the State of the Disorder. Such Kind of Evacuations proceed chiefly from a very great Corruption of Humours, the Violence of the Fever, or total Relaxation of the Fibres: Sometimes these Discharges are in too small a Quantity to be of any manner of Service, sometimes in too large a one for the Strength of the Patient to sustain, and sometimes their Matter is very bad; of this Class are Drops of black Blood, partial cold Sweats, bilious, acrid, greenish or black Stools, and Vomitings of the same Kind, such as frequently appeared in the Pestilential Constitution, and are often mentioned by Hippocrates to have happened at the Crisis of fatal Fevers.

... Moreover cutaneous Eruptions are undoubtedly to be classed with critical Abscesses.

... Hitherto I have endeavoured to explain whence acute Diseases have obtained so great a Variety of Names; what are the Signs of Crudity and Concoction; what the Tokens of Recovery, Danger, or Death; what the Presages of a Crisis; what Helps Nature herself makes use of for expelling a Fever; what Disorders each Evacuation is most suited to remove; and lastly, among those Evacuations and Abscesses, which are not critical, what are serviceable, what dangerous, and what fatal. I shall next proceed to the Method of curing acute Diseases: And here no one will deny, but Art must be directed so as to imitate Nature.

Commentary V
Of the Method of Diet in acute Diseases

The Diet in Fevers, ought to be neither too sparing or thin, nor on the other hand, too plentiful or substantial; for the Patients sink under the former, and are overcharged by the latter. We ought therefore to consult the Strength and Nature of the Disease, and Constitution and Way of living of the Patient, not only with regard to eating, but likewise drinking.

A moist and thin Diet is proper for all Persons in Fevers, but of this there are three degrees, viz. thin, exactly thin, and extremely thin.

Ptisan, or Barley Gruel is the thin; the Cream of Ptisan, or Barley Gruel strained, the exactly thin; and Water sweetened with Honey, or any other medicated Potion, containing no more Nourishment, is the extremely thin Diet: So that there are so many Sorts of moist and thin Diet, as there are different Degrees in the Acuteness of Fevers; and in general, one is accommodated to the other.

...Besides these Things. we ought to have a Regard to the Patient's Age, Constitution, Climate, and Custom, and likewise to the Season of the Year, and Symptoms of the Fever.

At this point Glass quotes from The Aphorisms:

With respect to Age, old Men; with respect to Constitution, those who are cold and phlegmatick, most easily bear Abstinence; but Children, especially the most lively, with the greatest Difficulty ...

He continues to expand on dietary details and modifications, appropriate to the type of fever, its severity and timing. It is no surprise to find frequent references to Hippocrates, himself such an ardent advocate of correctness in this matter, likewise Erasistratus, Chrysippus, Asclepiades, and Themison, founder of the Methodists, as related by Celsus:

But this part of Physick which relates to the curing of Diseases by Diet, is not attended to, with that Care it deserves, by those who are unac-quainted with the Observations of the Antients. Such, for the most Part, allow the same Food to all Persons, in all Kinds of Fevers, or, perhaps, enjoin nothing in this Case, but Abstinence from the grosser Kinds of Food, and so commit the whole Management of this Affair, to the Care of an old Nurse. And very few, indeed, are so sollicitous, as to make a Calculation of the Length of the Fever, that they may regulate the Diet thereby. But the same bad Symptoms, now adays as heretofore, are brought upon the Sick by improper Diet; though the generality of People do not perceive it; for such are not capable of distinguishing what Symptoms proceed from the Disease, what from the Physician, and what from the Patient; (to discover this, was a Talk worthy of Hippocrates:) So let what will happen amiss, or prove fatal, it is imputed to the Disease and its Malignity. And this is one of the crafty Devices Ignorance makes use of to keep itself concealed.

Commentary VI
Of Bleeding

Bleeding is of use in those Disorders where an Haemorrhage, happen-ing of its own accord, is beneficial. Now, in violent Fevers, when the Patient has Youth and Strength of [on] his Side, a Flux of Blood from the Nose, more frequently happens, and is of the greatest Service.

... But in these, and the like Circumstances, it is not to be left to Nature to bring on an Haemorrhage; because in acute Fevers , when the Patient is strong and full of Blood, there is much Danger of a great Inflammation, or perhaps of a Vessel's bursting about some of the more noble Viscera; which Evils are much more easily prevented, than remedied after they have happened: Besides, when there is any great Inflammation formed immediately at the Beginning of a Disease, it is much oftener brought to Suppuration, than dissolved by Nature; provided the Disease doth not kill the Patient before.

... Galen judged of the Patient's Strength, by the Pulse of the arteries, rather than by the Appearance of the Blood vessels; and if the Pulse was full and strong, he ordered Bleeding in the same Kind of Disorders: And all Physicians since his Time, have regarded this as a principal Indication for drawing Blood.

But when the artery lies deep, or the Patient's Breathing is difficult, ... this Sign is fallacious. It has besides a great many provisional Cautions, because the Arteries, as Celsus observes, treating of another Subject, move slower or quicker, according to the Difference of Age, Sex, and Constitution. And, generally, in a Person tolerably healthy, if his Stomach be out of Order; and sometimes, also at the first Attack of a Fever, the Pulse sinks and flags, so that a Man may seem to be weak, who has a violent Paroxysm coming on, which he is well able to bear. On the contrary, Fear, Anger, and any other Passion of the Mind, frequently quickens them: So that at the first Entrance of a Physician, the Patient's Concern what the Doctor may think of him, may possibly hurry his Pulse. For which Reason, a Physician ought not to seize his Patient by the Hand immediately, at his first coming in, but to sit down by him, and with a cheerful Countenance, enquire how he finds himself; and if he is under any Fear of Danger, to encourage him with proper Discourse, and then feel his Pulse.

... As to the Quantity to be taken away, that is to be regulated by the Habit of Body, the Season of the Year, the Age of the Patient and the Colour of the Blood. When all these are favourable, we ought, without Hesitation, to take away a larger Quantity: And if a violent Pain, about the superior Parts, together with an acute Fever, require Bleeding, we should bleed even to Fainting.

... And I have found, by manifold Experience, that this Remedy is of very great Service; for, by drawing off Blood, in very ardent Fevers, till the Patient faints, the whole Body is presently cooled, and the Fever extinguished: A great many hereupon fall into a gentle Looseness, and a Sweat; after which some immediately grow well, the others bear the Disease more easily, and recover in a little Time.

... The Antients used to open different Veins in different Diseases, with

a View of intercepting the Defluxion of Humours upon the Parts affected; or of drawing off the vitiated Juices from them. Herein, however, they disagreed, and there were some great Debates what particular vein should be opened almost in every Disorder. But this Contention is quite ceased since Harvey's Discovery of the Circulation of the Blood: And that vein which lies most convenient for the Lancet is now opened, except sometimes when, for the Sake of Derivation or Revulsion,[18] we chuse to bleed in the Jugular or Saphoena.

... Art hath found out yet another Method of drawing Blood, namely, by making Incisions in the Skin, and then applying Cupping Glasses. Hippocrates frequently made use of Cupping Glasses, both with and without Incision: When used without Incision, they were supposed to draw out Wind, and divert Defluxions. A Cupping Glass is mostly made use of when the Disorder does not equally affect the whole Body, but is fixed in some particular Part, the draining off the Humours from which, is sufficient to remove the Disease.

... Moreover, in acute Diseases, where the Disorder requires bleeding, and the Patient's weakness will not permit the opening of a Vein, Cupping is necessary; for this Remedy hardly sinks the Patient, and is never dangerous at any time in Fevers ...

Commentary VII
Of Purging and Vomiting

This is the longest commentary of all, extending to ninety pages, nevertheless Glass critically scanned the full range of Hippocratic writing and selected extracts for guidance:

We read in Hippocrates of some in Fevers who were gradually relieved, and others who were immediately cured by a Looseness. We know, likewise, that the Parent of Physick, copying after Nature, was frequently wont to purge in Fevers; and that after him the greatest Masters of the Art have approved of the same Remedy in the like Distemper ...

But he pointed out that attention was required to such a number of circumstances that no exact rules could be laid down concerning this method of cure, thus perhaps providing an escape route in the event of failure:

For it is no easy Matter, even for a skilful Practitioner, so to guide himself by his own Judgment, as not to err in Practice, and exceeding difficult to explain it in such a Manner, that others may not be led into Mistakes. For which Reason, he determined to leave it entirely to Physicians to acquire this Knowledge, by their own Practice and Observation. This great Man's Opinion almost deterred me from my

Design; but I was desirous of knowing, without hazardous Experiments, when Purging was required in Fevers. In order, therefore, to come at some Rules for purging, I carefully examined in what Circumstances of these Disorders, Hippocrates made use of this Remedy.

... If that bitter Humour, which we call yellow Bile, is collected in the Stomach, what Heat, Anxiety, and Faintness does it produce! Now, as soon as this Humour is discharged by a timely Evacuation, whether excited by Nature or Medicine, the Complaints vanish; but as long as it is retained, and remains crude and undigested, no Art can remove the Complaints, or put an end to the Fever. Moreover, if a sharp, acrid, greenish Humour infests the Stomach, what anguish of Mind, Dejection of Spirits, and acute Pains about the Thorax and Bowels, doth it occasion! Nor will these Complaints cease, till the offending Matter is purged and carried off, or corrected by being mixed with other Humours.

... The signs of turgid Matter about the Stomach are, universal Weariness, a sudden Weakness, Shiverings, a foul Tongue, a Bitterness in the Mouth, loathing of Food, Sickness at Stomach, uneasiness about the Praecordia, and Tumours of the same Part; which easily yield to the Pressure of the Fingers,

... Now all these bad Symptoms, and likewise the Fevers produced from the same Cause, cannot be removed by any Art, till the turgid Matter be sufficiently alter'd or expell'd by proper Evacuations. Therefore, according to the Precept of the greatest Master in Physick, when the Matter is turgid in the Beginning of Fevers, it must be purged off: If it has a Tendency upward, it is to be purged by Vomit; and if downward, by Stool; for the morbid Matter is to be carried off the nearest Way possible, provided it be a convenient one. Besides in this, we follow Nature as our Guide:

... Hippocrates was always afraid to bleed after Purging. 'Tis also equally bad to defer Purging till the Fever is become violent, and the Patient's Strength almost worn out by the Disease, and the Crisis at hand;

... Vomits likewise are given with greater Safety after Bleeding, when that is required. These ought to be given on the first Days.

... Purging is also very improperly used, where a Coldness of the Extremities presages an approaching Paroxysm. It is likewise very dangerous to those, where the Parts about the lower Belly are thin and emaciated; but in Diseases of the Breast, after digested Matter begins to be expectorated, it is fatal; for it puts a Stop to Expectoration, whereby the Patient, about the Time the Crisis was expected, is suffocated.

... When, therefore, it is judged necessary to give a Purge, and any of these Circumstances forbid Purging, we must have recourse to

Clysters. This Remedy is never dangerous;
... These gentle Methods are, 'tis true, safer than the more violent ones
used by the Antients. But then it must be consider'd, that as they are
attended with no Danger, so the Benefit received from them is less; nor
can a violent Disease be cured without as violent a Remedy.

The commentary contains an apparent digression on the *Colica Damnoniorum,* the Devonshire Colic, which it need hardly be said, is not a fever. Glass arrives here via a prolonged consideration of abdominal turgidity and biliousness in fevers. He was evidently struck by the epidemic nature of this illness, occurring every autumn on his own doorstep; moreover cold sweats were included among the violent symptoms which in some ways mimicked the onset of an acute fever. He quotes extensively from the essay on the Devonshire Colic, published in 1739, by John Huxham,[19] whom he describes as an 'Author who has greatly merited of his Country'. Huxham had painted a vivid clinical picture of lead poisoning, though it was not until 1767 that Sir George Baker made the connection between the colic, cider, and lead poisoning in that most remarkable piece of medical inductive reasoning.[20] Glass gives this as an example of a pituitous disorder and goes on to say:

That 'tis possible for this Matter to be corrupted, no one will deny, but
that from hence slow nervous Fevers are frequently produced, scarce
any one I believe will easily admit (because the hypothesis is new). But
the History of that Disease, and the Symptoms which accompany it,
have made it at least probable to me.

This indicates that Glass was privy to Huxham's concept of a 'slow nervous fever,' described in 1739.[21] It should be said that Huxham himself did not regard the Devonshire Colic in this category. Twentieth century experience reveals that one can indeed have a fever paradoxically without feverishness, where the infection is so overwhelming that the sufferer is cold and collapsed and in imminent danger of death. This is seen in, for instance, acute mengococcal septicaemia. Moreover, the regular seasonal outbreaks of the Devonshire Colic must have seemed very suggestive of a local epidemic of infectious illness. Slow fevers are thought to have been mainly typhoid, but also seem to embrace miliary fever and spotted fever.[22]

For slow Fevers are most frequent in Climates inclining to cold, in a
moist Constitution of the Air, and about damp marshy Places. They
visit those mostly, who are naturally weakly, or who are rendred so by
Grief or any other Accident; and also those who live upon a depraved
crude Diet ... The same Sort of people accustomed to the same Way of
living , particularly if subject to be costive, are particularly in Germany
afflicted with the miliary Fever. And 'tis very remarkable, that in
Scotland about Dumfries, when slow nervous Fevers were most
epidemical, not one was seized who lived well, and drank freely of Wine.

And very few besides the lower Class of People are seized with the spotted Fever which is now raging with us.

... In all, the Distemper daily affects the Head more and more, till at last they don't care either to speak or move, but are either excessively sleepy, or surprizingly watchful and restless; they talk madly; there's a subsultus of the Tendons, cold and inconstant Sweats, which sometimes are very profuse and clammy, and before their Death frequently very cold; they fumble about the Bedcloaths, and pick as it were Straws, and have a small creeping Pulse; at the last, perpetual cold Sighs indicate that Death is nigh.

... A plenty of red florid Pustules, or turgid miliary Eruptions appearing in the State of the Disease is a good Omen, ...sometimes when the first Crop of miliary Pustules is over, a second Eruption comes on, and this is sometimes repeated again and again, for the Space of several Weeks; then indeed the Fate of the Patient is very dubious.

... In this Disease likewise as in the colic before mentioned, the first Part of the Tragedy is acted about the Stomach by the corrupted Pituita.

There is a single reference towards the end of the commentary to the Boerhaavian concept of 'lentor', where the disease 'seems for the most Part to arise from a too great Disposition of the Blood to concrete'. It is to be treated by bleeding, followed by purging medicines.

Commentary VIII
Of Expectoration, and the Cure of an Inflammation of the Lungs, and a Pleurisy.

Glass repeats the Hippocratic teaching that where the lungs were inflamed it was to be expected that the disorder was to be carried off by an expectoration:

In the very beginning of these Disorders, or at least before the expectorated Matter is digested, we should bleed and purge the Patient as often as the Violence of the Fever, the Intenseness of the Pain and Inflammation, or the other Symptoms of the Disorder require. But when he begins to expectorate with ease well digested Matter, we should abstain from any considerable Evacuation whatever; notwithstanding, if the Fever runs too high, Hippocrates advises a Clyster to be thrown up now and then, in order to lower it.

... Therefore in a Peripneumony, as long as the Disease continues dry and violent, the Patient ought to be restrained from all Kinds of thicker Food, and even Spoon-meats; because such Sort of Diet will increase the Suffocation; for which Reason in this Disorder, the Diet should be extremely thin as in the most violent Fevers.

... As to Medicines, that which is composed of the Pine Cone, Galbanum and pure Honey, or any others of the like Virtue, are proper.
... The last Remedy in such a Disorder is a strong Vomit.

Mention is made of hot fomentations, either through a hot water bottle or a 'large soft Spunge taken out of hot Water and wrung'; there are instructions as to the making and use of a 'Vaporary' or inhalation. Finally:

Where the Pain of the Side continues violent, notwithstanding a suffi-cient Quantity of Blood has been drawn off, and other proper Remedies administred, we may have Recourse to Cupping with Scarification.

Commentary IX
Of the Discharge by Urine

A very short section which may be summarised in one paragraph:

But in order to carry off the acrid Salts, the urinous Oil, and the corrupted Serum, 'tis highly necessary in Fevers that the Urine should always pass off freely; for the the constant regular Passage assigned to those by Nature, is thro' the Kidnies; and these Feculencies are gener-ated in much greater Quantities in Fevers, than in Health ... If it be only therefore to wash off these Kinds of excrementitious Matter, larger Quantities of Liquids are required in Fevers than in perfect Health.

Commentary X
Of Sweating

It may be noted that Boerhaave's 'lentor' receives another mention in this commentary:

Sweat, or at least a gentle moisture of the Skin, is always to be wished for, towards the End of a Fever; for according to Hippocrates, acute Diseases are carried off either by the Mouth, or by Stool, or by Urine, or some such like Way, but Sweat is common to all.
... Now that which is evacuated by the Skin is the most subtile of all the Excrements of the Body, therefore the febrile Matter which is to pass off this Way ought to be exceedingly well attenuated and concocted, for which Reason critical Sweats generally succeed other Evacuations.
... Of all that immense Tribe of internal sudorific Medicines which have been brought into use by the Moderns, not one of 'em more certainly or with less Disturbance to the Body, promotes the Cutaneous Excretion, than Opium and Camphire mixed:
... some having observed, that almost all Fevers are terminated by

Sweat, and many of 'em (such as Fevers not lasting above a Day or two, and other slight ones arising from Errors committed with Regard to the six Non-naturals) are soon carried off by it, have imagined that Fevers of all Kinds are best cured by Sweating. Hence from the times of the Arabians, a great variety of sudorific Medicines began to come into use, which indeed we see given to all indiscriminately, immediately in the Beginning of Fevers, without any Regard to the Preparation of the febrile Matter.

... This great and vulgar Error of Physicians was strongly opposed by Sydenham, who not only rejected the use of hot sudorific Medicines in Fevers, as well as loading the Patients with a great many Cloaths, but wou'd have the Sweats which flow'd of their own Accord in the Beginning of the Disease, prevented.

... the Words of Sydenham, whose Judgment those great Lights of Physick, Mead, Friend, and Boerhaave, and many others of principal Note have confirm'd in their Writings. For those then who have the Care of the Health and Lives of their Fellow Creatures to despise Admonitions of such great Importance, is highly criminal, but knowingly to use a Method for protracting Diseases, in order to enrich themselves, is practising the Art of poisoning.

... When Sweats then are forced out by hot Medicines in the Beginning of Fevers, especially inflammatory ones, where a sizy 'lentor' of the Blood is a great Part of the Disorder, the vital Humour will be prodigiously thicken'd, and by that Means rendred unfit to circulate thro' the extreme capillary Arteries, but being impell'd with Violence, will be forced into them, and there stick fast.

... In slow Fevers also, where warm Medicines are wanted to quicken the vital Motion, we must take care that we are not too busy with them. How exceedingly pernicious hot alexipharmick Medicines are in the miliary Fever, Experience hath too frequently taught us;

... In the Plague therefore, a plentiful Profusion of Sweat, excited by hot Medicines, with the Allowance of a large Quantity of diluting Drinks, is the chiefest Remedy, if it be used before the Venom is obstinately fix'd on any particular Part. But this Method has been attempted in the Small Pox, with the loss of a great many Lives;

Commentary XI
Of the Cure of Critical Abscesses

If the abscess therefore is purely inflammatory, those things are to be apply'd to it, which will soonest bring it to Suppuration; for in ardent Fevers where tumours arise near the Ears, and do not suppurate, the Patients seldom recover. But where they suppurate with Signs of Concoction, and contain white Matter, they are salutary.

It seems he is probably referring here to an acute mastoiditis, just as he is evidently referring to an acute osteomyelitis in this:

> I had a Patient who was on a sudden freed from a malignant Fever by an Abscess in his Thigh whilst the Urine continued crude; the Thigh Bone from thence became carious, and the Lameness and Ulcer still remain, though this happen'd seven Months since.
>
> ... The Spots which appear in Fevers are seldom sufficient to receive all the morbid Matter, and oftentimes they come out without giving any Manner of Relief; hence some have imagined them to contribute nothing at all towards the Crisis of a Fever. But 'tis certain, that Spots have sometimes perfectly carried off this Disorder, and without any other assistance; and also that when they are thrown out either too soon or too late, it presages ill, but when they come out seasonably, good. wherefore I think the Petechiae ought to be ranked with critical Abscesses; however, for the most Part some other Assistance is wanted. The Petechial Fever is generally reckoned amongst malignant and mortal Diseases, and when treated according to Art, is easy to be cured, and a very safe Disease.

Specific instructions follow for the treatment of the Petechial Fever, including cleansing the stomach and intestines, bloodletting, before the eruption if possible. If indicated at a later stage, cupping glasses are to be applied to the neck with scarification; the motion of the blood is to be stimulated by opium and warm penetrating medicines but not in such a quantity as to raise a sweat. Inflammatory thickness of the blood is to be attenuated with nitrous medicines, a putrid dissolution is to be corrected with acids and astringents and a crude viscous 'lentor' by dissolving it with alkaline salts, exactly saturated with acids, and also with blisters. In the very late stages at the approach of the crisis a kindly sweat should be provoked.

With regard to abscesses, if there is no sign of a critical evacuation (or suppuration) then bleeding, purging and sweating are to be employed.

Commentary XII
Of Blisters

There is an initial review of the historical use of blistering agents of which cantharides was the only one to stand the test of time; mustard, pyrethrum and adarce are only briefly mentioned. In spite of the almost universal enthusiasm for the use of cantharides in fevers, from what is said later, Glass had some reservations:

> However, the Use of Blisters with Cantharides is very frequent among us at this Day, insomuch that there's hardly any dangerous Fever, where the Application of them is not by the Generality of Physicians

religiously observed. For these Reasons, a Physician ought to know what is to be expected from this Remedy, which indeed can be learned no other Way than by faithful Experiments.

A section follows in which some experiments by Baglivi are reported, involving the addition of cantharides to blood and the injection of it into the jugular vein of a dog; the rather horrific results of the latter are described in some detail.

The observations of Diascorides on the toxic effects of ingesting cantharides are quoted, with its drastic effects on the urinary organs; and he adds:

Besides these Symptoms, Physicians have sometimes observed enormous Priapisms to succeed the swallowing of Cantharides.

If priapism was a recognised side effect of cantharides poisoning, it no doubt gave rise to the often repeated myth of the aphrodisiac effects of Spanish Fly.

Glass then makes it very clear that there is equal toxicity when the substance is applied to the skin:

Upon the Application of Cantharides to the Skin in Fevers, the Thirst as well as Dryness of the Tongue is increased, the Pulse becomes more quick and frequent; but sometimes it is fuller, and sometimes more contracted, the Fever is hightened, and now and then the Bladder is tormented with lancing Pains, especially when fresh Blisters are applied to the ulcerated Parts before they are well covered with new Skin; sometimes Blood, and Pellicles like abraded Membranes are brought off with the Urine; and in those who have had such Symptoms, the Bladder has been found ulcerated after Death; the Discharge of Urine is generally increased, sometimes it is entirely suppressed, but more frequently made with Pain, and Drop by Drop.

... Since then in acute Fevers, a Delirium follows upon a Retention of those Salts which ought to be carried off through the Kidnies; since the Poison of Cantharides chiefly attacks the Head, next to the urinary Passages; and since Fevers attended with a Dissolution of the Blood are very apt to seize upon the Brain, it is not certain that Blisters are absolutely necessary in all Disorders of the Head and Nerves. On the contrary, in Fevers where the Blood is dissolved and acrid if Disorders of the Head threaten or have seized the Patient,'tis reasonable to think that Blisters will sooner bring them on, and more violently increase them. It is allowed even by those who so strenuously contend for the use of Blisters in all kinds of Fevers, that a Delirium and Subsultus of the Tendons have ensued, and increased on the Application of Blisters. Yet some have such a bigotted Opinion of their Virtue in these Disorders, that they persuade themselves, whatever bad Symptoms of this kind happen'd, entirely flowed from the Disease, and wou'd have been more violent if this Remedy had been omitted; but since these

74

*Symptoms sometimes come on soon after the Application of Blisters ...
I can never be induced to believe that Cantharides are an effectual
Remedy in all Disorders of the Head and Nerves.*

*... Now it is quite contrary to Reason to apply a strong Dissolvent to
the Blood, when it is already too much dissolved, and to exalt by Means
of a most acrid Salt, what hath already too great Acrimony, and to
irritate the Arteries with a violent Stimulus, when their Motion is
already immoderately quick and frequent. Yet all these things are to be
expected from the Use of Blisters in these Kinds of Fevers.*

There are, however, two or three indications that Glass allows:

*Wherefore, in Fevers which are inflammatory or rheumatick, or those
which happen in the Winter time, and others where the Blood drawn off
has a sizy Crust on its Surface like Glue, or Leather, or where it is too
thick, Blisters are of notable Service to dissolve this Lentour; but the
Arteries in inflammatory Fevers, have too violent a Motion; for which
reason this Remedy shou'd not be used till after proper Bleedings;
... In slow Fevers likewise, and in all those where the Pulse is too
languid for the Nature of the Disease, Blisters are of great Use to
quicken it.*

In the special case of smallpox, Glass quotes from a correspondence with John
Friend:

*One of the most celebrated Physicians of this Age, who hath by a long
Practice experienc'd the Virtues of Cantharides himself, and has
frequently seen what hath been done with them by others, says that
Patients in the small Pox (in which Disease there are some who never
omit Blisters, if the Disorder is violent) require Blistering when the
Fever is attended with a small and languid Pulse, and there's little or
no swelling of the Hands, and with a general Decay of Strength the
Patient is rather chilled than overheated.*

Finally, attention is drawn to the part played by blisters in treatment by revulsion:

*Thus a Blister to the Neck, is judg'd best to draw off Defluxions from
the Eyes, Fauces, and Windpipe; the same is apply'd to the Head or
behind the Ears, to make a Revulsion from the Brain; but when the
Humours are to be drawn from the middle Parts of the Body, we should
apply Blisters to the Extremities, and if the upper Parts are to be
relieved, blister the lower.*

Notes

(1)   W. Munk, *Western Times*, 1855, 13 October, p.8.   Dr Carter's annotations drew attention to inelegancies of diction at certain points, but the general tone was complimentary.   The particular note which Munk mentioned read

> *Utilissima sane sunt haec commentaria, et terlecta juvabunt; inter auctorem et meipsum olim intercedebat consuetudo. Boerhaavii ad pedes prima Medicinae elementa docuit, et vir est artis ipsius in primis peritus.*

(2)   G.E. Rehberger, *Lippincott's Quick Reference Book for Medicine and Surgery* (Philadelphia and London, 1940), p. 436b.

(3)   Thomas Sydenham, *Observationes Medicae* (1676).   Sydenham followed Hippocratic tradition in three main respects, in accurate clinical observation, in an epidemiological approach, and in an adherence to the Hippocratic doctrine of the humours.   See Kenneth Dewhurst, *Dr Thomas Sydenham* (London, 1966), pp. 60, 61.

(4)   Richard Mead, *The Medical Works of Richard Mead* (Edinburgh,1775), pp 159, 224, 347.   It is clear that Mead followed both Hippocrates and Sydenham.   In the case of smallpox and measles he made an additional valuable contribution by sponsoring the translation of the treatise of Rhazes, who also perpetuated Hippocratic teachings.

(5)   Friedrich Hoffmann (1660-1742), Professor of Medicine at Halle.

(6)   Georg Stahl (1660-1734), a brother professor at Halle.   He was a protagonist of *animism*, who explained life and disease by the action of a *sensitive soul*, or *anima*, which inhabited every part of the organism and prevented its spontaneous putrefaction. See Erwin.H. Ackerknecht, *A Short History of Medicine* (Baltimore and London, 1982) p. 128.   Fever in his hypothesis consisted in a *spasmus tonicus*.   Hoffmann followed up these ideas, omitting the metaphysical aspects and allowed a wider range and longer term to the constrictive spasm of fever, changing its name to *spasmus periphericus*.

(7)   John Huxham, *Observationes de aere et morbis epidemicis* 1728-1739, (London,1739). His essay on the Devonshire Colic was bound with this.

(8)   John Barker, *An inquiry into the nature, cause and cure of the present epidemick fever*, (London, 1742).

(9)   See G.E.R.Lloyd in *Hippocratic Writings* (Penguin Classics, 1986), p. 21 et seq.

(10)   R.Hooper, *Medical Dictionary* (London, 1831), p.573.

(11)   Ibid., p.573.   See also Lester S. King, *The Medical World of the Eighteenth Century* (Chicago, 1958), p. 83.

(12)   Saul Jarcho, introduction to *John Huxham, An Essay on Fevers*, (Watson Publishing International, 1988).

(13)   William Cullen, *First Lines of the Practice of Physic*, (New York, 1793), pp 4877.

(14)   William F. Bynum, 'Cullen and the study of fevers in Britain, 1760-1820,' *Medical History*, Supplement No. 1, 1981, pp 135-137. This gives a full account of Cullen's views on fevers.

(15)   Lester S. King, op. cit. note(10), p. 79.

(16)   Lloyd, op. cit., note (9) above, p.32.

(17)   The pythagorick numbers undoubtedly had a magical as well as a mystical significance and it is interesting to witness the gradual elimination of magical concepts, much of which happened in the eighteenth century. The number 'seven' was of special importance in that it formed a bond of union between body, soul and spirit on the one

hand and evil, disunion and strife on the other. See C.J.S.Thompson, *Magic and Healing* (London,1946) p. 164. This author pointed out that the seventh day was critical in all acute diseases.

(18)   Galen described the use of bloodletting in order to divert blood from a particular part of the body, the two methods being *derivation* and *revulsion*. See P.Brain, *Galen on Bloodletting*, (Cambridge, 1986), pp 13, 33, 129.

(19)   Huxham's essay on the Devonshire Colic was bound with his *Observationes de aere...*, see note (7) above.

(20)   See Sir George Baker, *An inquiry concerning the cause of the Endemial Colic of Devonshire* in The Medical Transactions of the College of Physicians (London 1785) p. 175, having been read at the college June 29, 1767. In his paper Baker quotes figures of admissions for the colic to the Devon and Exeter Hospital from 1762 to 1767, notified by Dr Andrew, p.200.

(21)   In Huxham's *Essay on Fevers* (1750) p. 72, he speaks of 'the very great difference between the putrid malignant and the slow nervous Fever ... Nor do I know any Author, that hath done it explicitly, besides Dr Langrish' (Browne Langrishe) in his *Modern Theory and Practice*, (London, 1738), pp. 329,331. His first mention of this was in *Observations de aere...* See note (7), above. See also R.M.S. McConaghey, John Huxham, *Medical History* 13 (1969), pp.280-287.

(22)   Spotted Fever has numerous synonyms. Although cerebrospinal fever (meningitis) has been socalled, see Sir William Osler, *The Principles and Practice of Medicine* (New York and London, 1912), p.108, the term is normally considered to apply to typhus, historically of much more significant epidemic importance. Other names for this disease were hospital or jail fever, petechial fever, and the common putrid or pestilential fever, see Osler, op. cit. p. 352 and Lester S. King, op. cit., note (10) above, p. 133; the condition was described notably by Sir John Pringle in his *Observations on the Diseases of the Army* (1752).

Miliary Fever is also known as the English sweating sickness, a very rapidly fatal illness in the 15th and 16th centuries, see Douglas Guthrie, *A History of Medicine* (London, 1958), p. 169; it died out in its original form, to reappear in 1718 in Northern France, being dubbed the 'Suette des Picards'. Osler, op. cit. p. 387, writing in 1912, mentions 'Within the past few years there have been several small outbreaks in Austria'.

Both miliary and petechial (i.e. spotted) fevers are discussed by Mead, op.cit. Note [4] above, pp. 349, 351. He agrees with Sydenham about the value of Jesuit's bark in the former, and in the latter, like Glass, condemns the practice of giving hot medicines in order to raise sweats, preferring the bezoardic powder or compound root of contrayerva.

Charles Creighton in *A History of Epidemics in Britain*, (2nd edition, London, 1965), Vol.II, p.128, implies that miliary fever was not an entity in itself. In many cases the miliary lesions were induced by treatment, or they were manifestations of other fevers, such as typhus.

CHAPTER V
Samuel Glass and the Magnesia Alba Fracas

Born in 1715, Samuel was the eldest of Thomas's three younger brothers who survived childhood. He was apprenticed to the surgeon apothecary Nicholas Peters, friend and associate of his brother, who lived at Topsham, the seaport at the mouth of the Exe, and who is referred to elsewhere. The apprenticeship commenced in 1729 and lasted five years,[1] following which Samuel set up as a surgeon apothecary in Oxford.

A number of years before, and almost certainly prior to 1748,[2] Thomas had discovered a way of making Magnesia Alba (magnesium carbonate), a useful and effective medicine for dyspepsia, and still, today the basis of many proprietary remedies. Unlike other preparations of magnesia, which were gritty, chalky, of variable purity, and with an unpleasant taste, his was a pure, exceptionally light powder, and quite tasteless.

In due course Thomas passed the details of the process over to his brother, who began to make it, at first in a small way, but later when the demand became established, as a commercial enterprise; its success prompted Samuel, in 1764, to publish *An Essay on Magnesia Alba*. In this he says:

> *The first insight I had into the process for preparing Magnesia I owe entirely to my brother, which he communicated to me as a matter of mere speculation and amusement. To see two equally pellucid liquors, upon mixing them together, form a white coagulum; to see this immediately dissolve upon pouring on it some boiling water, and the milky liquor in a short time deposit a white powder, was both new and curious. To be informed that this was the Magnesia Alba mentioned in a pamphlet, just then published, on the nursing and management of children; to hear that this powder was not generally known to the Faculty in England, but would prove a valuable acquisition to the Materia Medica, and be of great service in practice, was instructive and entertaining. And here perhaps the matter might have rested, had not the utility of the medicine been mentioned, and its use recommended, to that judicious and indefatigable Physician, the late Doctor Pitt of Oxford; who ... prevailed on me to prepare a little for him, by the process that had been communicated to me, as none was at that time to be had in the shops. The success which attended the use of it far exceeded his expectations; ... it was not long, however, before he renewed his application and observed, that the powders sold under the name of Magnesia were, both in their appearance and effects, very*

different from each other, and from that which I had prepared. ... That
he might rely therefore on the due preparation of the medicine, and do
justice to his patients, he advised those, in whose cases he thought the
powder would be serviceable, to send for it to my house.

True to his time, Samuel did not let slip the opportunity of mentioning the
patronage he had received from the nobility, including Lady Charlotte Finch,
governess to the Prince of Wales, who had ordered magnesia on behalf of the
royal infant.

In the course of thirty-eight pages, there is a careful review of the various
chemical processes used to produce this substance, and a diverse historical
parade of the chemists and physicians that devised them; names such as Van
Helmont, Hoffmann, Lancisi, and more recently Dr Black of Edinburgh. He
quotes at length from Dr Cadogan's essay *On the Nursing and Management of
Children:*[2]

> *at the first appearance of predominating Acid, which is very obvious*
> *from the green stools, gripes, and purgings occasioned by it. The*
> *common method, when these symptoms appear, is to give the Pearl*
> *Julep, Crab's Eyes, and the Testaceous Powders; which though they do*
> *absorb the Acidities, have this inconvenience in their effect, that they*
> *are apt to lodge in the body and bring on a costiveness, very detrimen-*
> *tal to infants, and therefore require a little Manna, or some gentle purge*
> *to be given frequently to carry them off. Instead of these I would recom-*
> *mend a certain fine insipid powder, called Magnesia Alba ... I have*
> *taken it myself, and given it to others for the heartburn and find it to*
> *be the best and most effectual remedy for that complaint.*

There is no doubt that Samuel derived a considerable income from the manufacture of this medicine and that the secret, being valuable, was jealously
guarded. He died in 1773 ,and perhaps it was with a sense of impending
dissolution that he sold out to a Peter Delamotte,[3] for a sum of one thousand
five hundred pounds, excluding utensils in his laboratory, stock and fixtures,
in April 1772.

There were, as it happens, others who had cast covetous eyes on this little
gold mine, in particular one Thomas Henry, who fourteen years previously
had worked as a journeyman to Mr Marlbon, an Oxford apothecary in the
neighbourhood of Samuel Glass, and was now established in Manchester,
where he was busy making Magnesia Alba, having had some 'useful hints'
about Mr Glass's methods.

No sooner had Samuel sold out than Henry, with a double-pronged attack,
attempted to corner the market in Magnesia. Firstly he wrote *An Account of
An Improved Method of making Magnesia Alba,* which he managed to get
published by the Royal College of Physicians in the second volume of their
Transactions, thus implying, incorrectly, that the College had given him its

patronage; secondly, in 1773, by which time Samuel was dead, he tried to destroy Delamotte, by stating that his powder was grossly inferior to that of his late master, furthermore it was more expensive; these allegations were contained in an appendix to his main essay, reprinted in *Experiments and Observations*, entitled *Strictures on Mr. Glass's Magnesia*.[4]

Henry began by criticising Samuel's essay because it said no more than that which everyone knew already, that Magnesia was made from Epsom salts and pot ashes and imputed meanness that no more detail was supplied. The common eighteenth century tactic was adopted by Henry, whereby his essay was dedicated in fulsome terms to an eminent Manchester physician, Thomas Percival.[5] Percival, himself, does not appear to have entered into the controversy at this stage, in fact he may have been somewhat embarrassed by his involvement, since he was strongly of the opinion that medical disputes should be referred to arbitration and not made public.[6] On the whole, however, Henry was fairly restrained in his criticism of Samuel's powder, content with the statement that his own was equal and in some respects better. He does in passing make one rather revealing observation:

> *Happening some years ago to live in the neighbourhood of a gentleman who has long been celebrated as the preparer of the most genuine Magnesia, and never having been able myself to make Magnesia comparable to his, by the commonly known methods, I was desirous of gaining some intelligence as to his process, and was at last so fortunate as to obtain some useful hints.*

Needless to say the gentleman concerned was Samuel Glass. The *Strictures*, published eighteen months after the first paper, are a different matter and Henry, very conscious of the affront he was causing, began:

> *It is with the utmost reluctance I find myself indispensibly obliged to address the public on a subject, from the nature of which I may perhaps incur the suspicion of acting from interested views...*

He then gave another little puff to the publication of his paper by the Royal College and went on to heap obloquy on Delamotte and his version of Glass's powder, and, incidentally, to advertise where his own powder was to be obtained.

Delamotte, fighting for his livelihood, came back with spirit in *A Refutation of Mr. Henry's Strictures on Glass's Magnesia*;[7] in this he enlisted the help of four eminent members of the Faculty in the University of Oxford, who carried out tests on both Glass's and Henry's products and found the former invariably of much greater purity. The experts involved were Doctors Smith, Vivian (Regius Professor of Physic), Parsons, and Wall:

> *In February, 1773, Mr. Glass died, and immediately Thomas Henry, ... observing with envy the universal esteem in which Glass's Magnesia*

was held, and long desirous of wresting to himself so beneficial a branch
of commerce, avails himself of this opportunity, and publishes what he
entitles Strictures on Glass's Magnesia.

... After having thus imposed upon the College of Physicians, and after
his Veracity had been found to be as light, as his Magnesia was heavy,
by every man who had a pair of scales in his possession.

... a few simple obvious proofs are sufficient to determine the whole
controversy, and let Mr. Henry change about, shuffle, scribble, prate,
puzzle, and bamboozle ever so much he will not be able to get over them,
in the opinion of the judicious reader.

The subject has already been taken up by Dr Glass, Physician of Exeter,
a Gentleman whose distinguished abilities are too well known in the
literary world for me to presume a word in his commendation. I dare
only embrace this opportunity of expressing my great obligations to
him, for the generous declaration he has been pleased to make in regard
to my reputation and property...

... happy had it been for my Opponent, had either his Modesty, his
Diffidence, or a sacred regard for Truth restrained him within the
bounds of Decency. And doubtless he merits this Admonition, That
however his Avarice or his Necessities might plead, the attempt of grat-
ifying the one or relieving the other at the Expence of my Reputation
and Fortune, was not only mean, but criminal.

There is a series of nine letters still existing from Delamotte to Thomas Glass, between June 1773, and January 1774:[8] they betray considerable anxiety and agitation as well as an obsequious attitude to the recipient. They seek advice, reassurance, and report the actions taken to deal with Henry's allegations; for instance:

Oxford, 19th June, 1773

Dear Sir

Your much esteemed Favour came duly to Hand. Since my last I have
the Pleasure of informing you that Dr Parsons, Professor of Chymistry
here has made Experiments on my Magnesia and finds it entirely free
from Mr. Henry's assertions. Dr Smith and the rest of the Gent. of the
Faculty are quite ready to assist me and all agreed at a Meeting that he
is a mere Quack and that an Action for Damages ought to be brought
against him...

Would you not think it advisable, Sir, to answer Mr. Henry without
waiting the Event of a Suit at Law? I yesterday received an order from
Mrs.Floud.

I am, with much esteem and respect, Dr Sir,
Your obliged humble servant P.Delamotte.

At the end of Delamotte's *Refutation*, by way of a testimonial, he appends a letter from John Huxham, who had died in 1768. The letter had been sent to Samuel, prompted by the gift to Huxham of a box of Magnesia, accompanied by his pamphlet on that subject. The letter was sent from Plymouth on May 18, 1764:

> *Sir*
>
> *I received your polite letter, ingenious dissertation, and very kind present last week; for which I very heartily thank you*
> *Your Magnesia is greatly superior in lightness, brightness, smoothness, and goodness to any I have ever seen from abroad or at home.*
> *I could never make any so beautiful and light, tho' I most carefully washed the Precipitate in many waters, hot and cold, and boiled it both in fresh water and oystershell lime water, in order more perfectly to divest it of the vitriolic salts and I then dried it with a pretty strong heat; yet none of mine was equal to yours.*
> *'Tis but doing justice therefore to your Preparation to recommend it strongly to the Public on all proper occasions; which I shall not fail of doing: and particularly have this very day desired two Ladies of distinction, who are for the moment under my care, to send for some of it for their use as soon as they return to Bath. I have given them a specimen of your's.*
> *I have at present an inflammation in my eyes, that makes writing troublesome to me, otherwise I might have said more on this head, but can now only assure you that I am, Sir,*
> *Your greatly obliged,*
> *And most obedient Servant*
> *J. Huxham.*

The letter had no doubt been amongst Samuel's belongings when Delamotte took over his establishment.

This was by no means the end of the dispute, which continued like a rather ponderous game of tennis, the initiative next being taken by Thomas Glass,[9] Henry responding in defence.[10]

Thomas Glass made it clear that the task of replying to Henry's Strictures was a very disagreeable one, but that it was undertaken to prevent the public from being deceived and Delamotte from being injured in his reputation and property, by Henry's false assertions and illiberal practices.

Reviewing his own part in the story, Thomas mentioned that he had communicated his discovery to several acquaintances, among them Mr (later Dr) Shebbeare who had supplied Dr Cadogan prior to the latter's *Essay on the Nursing and Management of Children*, published in 1748. He continued with a criticism of Henry:

> *after his process had been published by the College, and the Magnesia, he had produced, came to be sold at Mr Johnson's in St. Paul's*

Churchyard, any one, by taking up a box of it in his hand, might certainly know, that what Mr. Henry affirmed of its lightness, was an absolute falsehood. And he then found himself necessitated to acknowledge, that the Magnesia he produced was not equal to Mr. Glass's in lightness.

... But Mr Henry, whose view and design, whatever disinterestedness he may pretend, plainly is to ruin the credit of Glass's Magnesia, that he may introduce the sale of his own, assures the Public that he has discovered the amazing light Magnesia, now sold under the name of Mr. Glass, to contain no inconsiderable quantity of calcareous earth.

Thomas then went on to describe a series of detailed experiments which he had made to disprove Henry's allegations. Ingenious is a term of approbation often applied to eighteenth century medical and scientific figures, when Thomas referred to 'that ingenuous Apothecary from Manchester' it seems that the gentle pun had a more pejorative meaning than the word would have today. He is however most scornful of Henry's action in inducing:

the College of Physicians to publish his account in their Transactions; and make this a pretence to advertise in his bills, that his process for making Magnesia has been honoured with the patronage of that Learned Body.

Henry's attack on Delamotte had evidently rebounded on himself, for he refers in his *Letter to Dr Glass* to:

the illiberal abuse which I have suffered, for some weeks past, in almost every newspaper in the kingdom; after being publickly held up, as a malicious and interested obtruder of falsehood and detraction; it was with a mixture of deference and pleasure, I was informed, by an advertisement, that the ingenious and learned author of the Commentaries on Fevers had resolved to wield his pen against me.

He reacted to Glass's *Examination* with apparent pained surprise, it was evidently not what he expected of a physician and a gentleman. He mentioned that it was his friend, Dr Percival, who had approached Dr Warren, Physician to his Majesty, to read the paper at the College.

Most of the letter is a wordy repetition of what had been said wordily already; he could not resist an occasional malicious dig at Peter Delamotte, 'the ingenious stationer from Weymouth, with all his extraordinary fund of chemical knowledge'.

He returns, in between his rather waspish sallies, to his wounded *amour propre*:

Under the, almost unexampled, torrent of abuse which has so rapidly flowed upon me, the mens conscia recti, has been my great consola-

tion, and the citadel, from which I have calmly looked down on these feeble, though invidious attacks,

Nil conscire sibi, nulla pallescere culpa. *[He who is conscious of no guilt will not grow pale when accused.].*

There was, however, one muted apology; the fact that the College had published his paper had, he owned, given him the right to assume that they had given him their approbation. Either his agent or the printers had changed the word approbation for patronage in the first advertisements; this was done without his authority.

In spite of Percival's general unwillingness to become embroiled in a public slanging match, Henry managed to extract from him a character reference, which in the form of a letter from Percival to himself was added as an appendix:

Though it gives me great pain, dear Sir, to interfere in your dispute with a physician of deserved eminence in the literary world, who has honoured me with his correspondence, and, I flatter myself, with a share in his friendship, I cannot refuse my consent to the publication of the paper, which you have in your possession. For however I may respect and esteem Dr Glass, justice and truth have a superior claim to my regard, and lay me under an indispensable obligation to confirm, as far as my evidence can have any weight, your strictures on Mr. Delamotte's Magnesia ...

Glass and Percival therefore found themselves on opposite sides and perhaps the whole matter was never finally resolved, other than by the forgiving hand of time.

Bound with Thomas Glass's various tracts on this affair, is one more, by 'A Physician', undated, and entitled *Remarks on Mr. Thomas Henry's Improved Method of preparing Magnesia Alba.* Dealing largely with the chemical principles involved, in the space of sixty-two pages, it deals with the claims of both sides, which the author describes as:

a tiresome controversy, between the Oxford and Manchester preparers of this article, very disinteresting to the community in general ...

He called a plague on both their houses, in fact, but is on the whole much more critical of Henry, whose essay: 'affords us no exalted idea of his chemical genius'.

For good measure he describes yet another and better process for producing elegant Magnesia Alba, as well as one, derived from Dr Black, appearing in the Edinburgh Pharmacopeia. In the latter part of the appendix to his essay he mentions that the work was nearly completed when:

an advertisement appeared in one of the public papers, observing that Mr. Henry's manner of preparing Magnesia Alba had been read before the College of Physicians, and was inserted in the Medical Transactions.

... The College candidly declare they do not as a body, mean to vouch for the truth of any relation; or to give authority to any opinion, contained in their papers.

The author indulges in a final digression on the place of Magnesia Alba in the treatment of that very pressing problem of the eighteenth and nineteenth centuries, that 'of stones in the bladder and kidnies' [sic]. Standard treatment was the 'soap ley'. Investigation was required into whether magnesia had itself a lithontriptic virtue or whether, as some maintained, it interfered with conventional treatment.

The reputation of Glass's magnesia lasted well into the nineteenth century; an advertisement in the *Sheffield Iris*, April 27, 1830 reads:

The Magnesia prepared from the recipe of the late Dr Glass is the purest and most freed from saline and heterogeneous particles of any magnesia now made. Mr Delamotte last year assigned all his interest in the above property to E.Edwards, chymist, 67, St. Paul's Church yard ...[11]

Thomas Henry (1734-1816) became a well-known figure in Manchester Society, accumulated considerable wealth, and founded a dynasty bound closely to his Magnesia business, earning him the nickname 'Magnesia Henry'. One of his sons, William, and a grandson, William Charles, were physicians at Manchester. He was elected FRS in 1775 and was in at the beginning of the Manchester Literary and Philosophical Society (the 'Lit and Phil') in 1781. His son William wrote a memoir of his father, and acknowledged his hot temper, as witness the lack of amiability shown in his controversies with Glass and Delamotte. It has been suggested that he might have suffered from mercury poisoning, to which many apothecaries were prone. His handwriting, it is said, in middle age was tremulous and 'elderly', but improved after his retirement. Both personality and muscular control are affected by mercury poisoning, recovering when contact ceases.

The firm of T. & W. Henry was actively engaged in the manufacture of magnesia until 1933, when it was sold to British Drug Houses.[11]

Notes

(1)   See P.J. and R.V. Wallis, *Eighteenth Century Medics*, (Newcastle, 1988).

(2)   In Thomas Glass, *An Examination of Mr. Henry's Strictures on Glass's Magnesia*, (London, 1774), p.6, it is stated that his discovery was made prior to 1748, when Dr William Cadogan (1711-1797) published his *Essay on the Nursing and Management of Children*, London, 1748).

(3)   According to Henry, Delamotte was a stationer from Weymouth.

(4)   Thomas Henry, *An Account of an Improved method of preparing Magnesia Alba*,

(London, 1773). This was published first in *Med. Trans. Roy. Coll. Physicians*, **2**, 226-34, 1772, reprinted in *Experiments and Observations* ... (London, 1773). along with five other essays, in which for good measure Henry aims a sideways blow at another of his rivals in the magnesia business, Mr. Dale Ingram, as well as many complimentary references to his hero, Dr Thomas Percival. *The Strictures on Mr. Glass's Magnesia* were published as an appendix to the reprint.

(5)   Thomas Percival was a well-known physician in Manchester, he was a pupil and friend of William Cullen, having graduated MD at Edinburgh. He was a FRS and a friend and collaborator of John Haygarth, John Fothergill and others of that group. He wrote *Medical Ethics*, (Manchester, 1803) and other works of importance.

(6)   See David Harley, 'Honour and property, the structure of professional disputes in eighteenth century English medicine', *The medical enlightenment of the eighteenth century*, (Cambridge, 1990), p.157.

(7)   Peter Delamotte, *A Refutation of Mr Henry's Strictures on Glass's Magnesia*, (Oxford, 1774). Delamotte's name did not appear on the title page, merely 'the present Proprietor of Glass's Magnesia'.

(8)   Devon Record Office, Reference 72/1/2/1. Quoted by permission of the Devon & Exeter Institution.

(9)   Thomas Glass, *op. cit.*, note 2.

(10) Thomas Henry, *A Letter to Dr Glass, containing a reply to his examination of Mr. Henry's Strictures...*, (London, 1774)

(11) See Juanita G.L. Burnby, A Study of the English Apothecary 1660-1760, *Medical History*, Supplement No. 3, (Wellcome Institute for the History of Medicine, 1983), 70n. This has a short biographical account of Thomas Henry, 70, 71.

A fuller memoir of his father by William Henry is in *Manchester Memoirs*, **3**, 204-40, 1819. A modern account of the family is provided by W.V .Farrar, K.R. Farrar, and E.L. Scott, 'The Henry's of Manchester', Parts IVI, *Ambix*, 20 (1973) 24 (1977).

   The suggestion that Henry suffered from mercury poisoning appears as a note in *Ambix*, 20, 207.

CHAPTER VI
Samuel and Oxford

The premium for Samuel's five-year apprenticeship to Nicholas Peters was £100. He was fourteen when he started, on November 8, 1729, and thus he completed his time in 1734, two years after his father, Michael, had died. Thomas now returned to Tiverton from Leyden.[1] There is no record of when he went to Oxford, setting up as a surgeon apothecary, but it was certainly prior to November 1746, for in that year he sent a clinical report of some interest to Dr Richard Mead, who presented it at a meeting of the Royal Society. The case concerned a young woman of twenty-four, who had suffered from an *An uncommon Dropsy from the Want of a Kidney...* and is set out as an appendix to this chapter.[2]

The next recorded event was on May 16, 1752, when Samuel Glass, surgeon, was granted priveleged status by the University, thus giving him authority to 'trade' within the University precincts.[3]

The prisoners in Oxford Prison, then euphemistically known as Oxford Castle, were evidently within the ambit of his practice, for he is recorded as having attended several inmates between February and July, 1753, these included: Greening (mortification in leg); Cormine (foul distemper); Forster (swelling in knee) and Medcroft (swelling in arm). His fees for this were £6.15s.6d. Bleeding the prisoners was evidently done by William Dennis, who earned 11s.6d. for bleeding four prisoners from October to June of that year; he was probably a barber. Samuel's name appears again in 1757, when he earned £7.2s. for attending six inmates. No diagnosis was given, merely a note that they were either debtors or felons.

In 1758 there were two patients: Evans (ulcers) 21s.; Guest, a debtor, (inflammation of the eye) 42s.

The work was clearly not very exacting, since again only two patients were noted in 1759: Watch (abscess) 7s.6d.; Lawrence (ulcer from 'the bite of an other man') 15s. The last two entries were for 1760 and 1761, respectively: Gloucester (rupture) 10s.6d. and Cowden (inflammation of the eye) also 10s.6d.[4]

It seems that by 1754 Samuel was now established in Oxford, since his lease of a house from University College started in this year. This was No. 33 High Street, directly opposite the college gates. The house was sold to Magdalen College in 1885, and by it to Queen's College in 1908; in 1936 it was incorporated with neighbouring houses into residential accommodation for Queen's College, the whole known as Drawda Hall; the downstairs part, fronting the street, are let as shops and retain the original street numbering. The house was one of University College's earliest investments, in about 1280. Samuel paid rent of 16s.8d. per annum.[5]

In 1754 also, Samuel himself took an apprentice; this was John Bulley, the period was for seven years and the premium £105.[6]

Samuel never married. In fact of all his brothers and sisters, Thomas was the only one who did. When he died, aged 58, he was relatively wealthy and able to leave various properties to his relatives. He left no correspondence or journal and no written work, other than his *Essay on Magnesia Alba* and the report on *An uncommon Dropsy...* . He was evidently on very good terms with his brother, Thomas, and figures in the marriage settlement of his eldest neice, Mary;[7] his other neices, Melony and Ann, were not married until after his death and Elizabeth never married. Samuel nevertheless remains a shadowy and enigmatic figure, drifting in and out of focus. Perhaps there is more to be learned by consideration of his will and the inventory of his house, than otherwise, in the way that the impression of a fossil creature may be discovered where it has lain.

Jackson's *Oxford Journal* printed an obituary, which indicates that Samuel had retired early, at least from surgical practice, presumably because he derived adequate income from his magnesia enterprise:

> *On thursday morning died, after a short illness, occasioned by a paralytic stroke, aged about 57, Mr Samuel Glass, late an eminent surgeon of this city, who had declined practice some years. He was a man of acknowledged skill and genius in his profession, of strict integrity, of a frank, liberal disposition, steady in his attachments, and hospitable to his friends: Hence his memory will be justly revered, whilst his loss is deservedly lamented.[8]*

Samuel still owned property in or near Tiverton, at Chevithorne, Sholimore, and Mere and a halfshare in an estate at Kitterbury. His brother Michael, his cousin Thomas, and his nephew John Vowler Parminter all benefited from their disposal.

The other Oxford house that Samuel rented belonged to Oriel College; it was a farmhouse, known as St Bartholemew's or Bartlemas, part of a small complex of buildings, the site of a twelfth-century leper hospital; this later became an almshouse, reverting temporarily to use as a hospital during the 1833 Oxford cholera epidemic; it is now privately owned. Alongside stands the perfectly preserved chapel, more than ever a place of tranquillity, just away from the turbulent Cowley Road.

The farmhouse is also still occupied, having been sold for private use in 1980. It was at Bartholemew's that the magnesia was made. The college leased the property to Samuel, with 15 acres of land, for 40s. per annum (money 26s.8d., corn 13s.4d.) and a couple of good fat capons on New Year's Day. His other obligation was to keep an ale house or victualling house in the said demised messuage, and from time to time during term, keep good and wholesome bread, beer or ale there, to be sold whereby the Almoners of Bartholemew's may have bread, beer and drink there, at reasonable rates.[9]

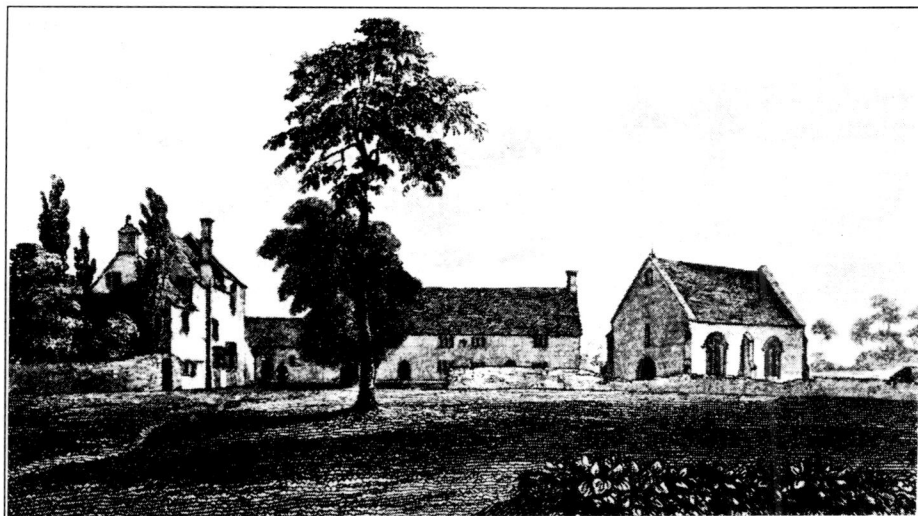

*Bartlemas. Farmhouse, almshouse and chapel in 1833,
from the engraving by G. Hollis.*

Samuel had an 'undertenant' or bailiff at Bartlemas by the name of Thomas Styles; to him he left a year's rent, all the tools for husbandry and gardening, excluding any thing used in the making of magnesia, a cart and the black horse, commonly known as Tetbury; his interest in both Oxford properties were left to his sisters, Mary and Elizabeth, still living in Tiverton. His youngest brother, Peter, had already died at the age of thirty-four, but he left £200 to his 'honoured' mother and the same to each sister and his brother, Michael; his servant, Joan Stool, received £5 and there was a guinea each to six poor men who should carry him to his grave. A codicil to the will was added on June 4, 1772, following the sale of the magnesia business, whereby the sum of £2000 was left on trust, benefiting first his sisters and brother, Michael, and then, after their deaths, his neices. Thomas was sole executor and was left the residue.[10]

The house in the High Street had five bedrooms, a dining room, hall, surgery, well-stocked kitchen, and a 'back house'; the latter is in fact a very substantial building, known nowadays as Little Drawda, and looks out on to the 'Nun's Garden', to be reached from the back of Queen's College. This explains the large amount of furniture allocated to this building in the inventory, which included five bedsteads (two being four-posters), a mahogany dining table and much else; lastly there was a brew house and a cellar. An inventory and valuation of the contents of the house was made at the request of Mr Delamotte by Richard Holloway, on March 8, 1773; the entire contents valued at £129.17.0. In the cellar were seventeen and a half dozen quart wine bottles at 2 shillings per dozen, and three dozen quart beer bottles at 18 pence per dozen, besides these were two hogsheads, two half hogsheads, seven kill-dorkins and a tap tub. Bearing in mind that Samuel kept an ale house at Bartholemews, it is tempting to relate Samuel's rather early demise to the generous contents of his cellar. Samuel's bedroom contained two large barometers and a smaller one, perhaps indicating an interest in climatology.[11]

There were problems, as it happened, with the house in Oxford High Street which mainly affected William Wickham, occupant of the neighbouring house, number 34, and Peter Delamotte. Wickham acted in certain respects as a local agent for Thomas Glass and a number of letters from him are still extant.[12] On May 12, 1775, he wrote to Thomas:

> I am sorry to acquaint you that the perpendicular spout between your house and mine, that carries off the water from Mr. Glass's house, which is brought down in an angle, made by the projection of my house, is so small, that a very little matter of filth stops it, when the water overflows and spreads and does great damage to your house and mine. My house was so much damaged by the same cause before that the corner post of my house was so perished that three parts in four of it was rotted through and became touchwood ...

Numbers 33 and 34 High street are still separated at street level by a narrow passage, and it is easy to picture the nuisance caused by a leaking downpipe. In a letter to Thomas on June 14, 1773, about magnesia, Delamotte writes as follows:

> I am obliged Sir to trouble you on the Subject of the House at Oxford____ You recollect the House of Office down the Yard, that, Sir, has no underground Reservoir for the Soil, but it goes into the Dung Hole; Mr. Wickham informs me the Commissioners will not allow this to be emptyed into the Street every 3 or 4 Months, (which the Dung Hole will not hold for longer), it being such a Filthy Jobb, and so offensive to the Neighbourhood, tho' taken up directly____ In Order to save you the Expence of digging of a Hole for the Soil, Mr Wickham & Self proposed (if agreeable to you) to take these Materials, & fitt up a former one, that has a large Under Ground Reservoir already, & that stands much more privater than the present, but is gone quite to Decay, not having been Used many years, it is in the little yard to the left Hand just before you come to the other. I did not know there was one there till last Week____Your Sense on this Matter also I begg to know.

Delamotte had his own problems with his health. On April 10, 1773, Wickham wrote to Mary Glass, the eldest of Samuel's two sisters:

> Last Night I received Dr Glass's letter with that part of the College Lease that you and your sister signed and this morning the Man that was sent for the Mare came here. Mr Delamotte is now very ill, he's

been eight days very dangerously ill and in exquisite pain by an infla-
mation in the Neck of his Bladder having no water passed till last night.
If his Disorder does not return We hope he is out of danger ...[13]

This was before Delamotte's intensive correspondence with Thomas about the magnesia problem, which began on June 19, 1773. Later, Delamotte evidently consulted Thomas about another medical matter for he wrote to him from Weymouth on November 22, 1776, and adds the following post-script: 'I have not yet gott rid of the violent heat and Itching in the Rectum, that I can get no Rest, many nights together.'[14] Delamotte was perhaps of a persistently anxious frame of mind and today's medical views would probably link this with his symptoms.

In the correspondence between Wickham and Thomas there are references to three Russian students, Messrs Nikitin, Bikoff, and Suvoroff, who owed Samuel money. In view of Samuel's roomy house it seems likely that they received board and lodging as well as tuition. They were still about in Oxford two years after Samuel's death and Wickham had some difficulty in getting them to pay their debts; it is even suggested that they threatened to claim the protection of the Russian Ambassador. In the end it was all settled, with the possible exception of a disputed £10, which occasioned a personal appeal from Basil Nikitin to Thomas.[15]

There was another Oxford resident who acted as an agent for Thomas Glass in business matters, this was Sackville Parker, a bookseller, opposite Queen's College in the High Street. He wrote in July 1781, to send his condolences on the death of Thomas's brother, Michael, so soon after the death of his unmar-ried daughter, Elizabeth. The last letter, of January 25, 1783, is melancholy and in part a request for medical assistance:

> *May this find Dr Glass and his Family in perfect Health___As to*
> *Myself, 'tis a Blessing I can by no Means boast of, I suspect having had*
> *a Parallitic Stroke, my limbs being greatly weakened, tho' not entirely*
> *lost: My heaviest Complaint is Want of Sleep, to procure which, I have*
> *too frequently had Recourse to composing draughts, which the next day*
> *so stultify, that I am quite tir'd of them: They likewise, almost totally*
> *destroy my Appetite: I wish therefore, that my Friend Dr Glass, wou'd*
> *favor me with a Prescription less prejudicial than that I have*
> *mention'd, but which may procure me the Blessing of Sleep___*

There is a footnote at the end: 'I scarcely think I shall ever be able to transact this business again.'[16] This was the year that saw the death of Thomas's wife, Mary.

Notes

(1)   See P.J. and R.V. Wallis, *Eighteenth Century Medics*, (Newcastle, 1988).
(2)   The Philosophical Transactions (1743-1750), abridged, (London, 1756), p. 1027.
And M.S., Wellcome Historical Medical Library, Ref. 2391/11 78820

(3)   Joseph Foster, Alumni Oxoniensis, 1715-1886, p.528.

(4)   Oxfordshire Quarter Sessions records, 1687-1830, 1754 T9; 1757 T10; 1762 Ep.7.

(5)   University College (Oxford) Archives, General Account Book D.

(6)   P.J. and R.V. Wallis op. cit.

(7)   Marriage settlement of Mary Glass, DRO, 49/9/6/213

(8)   Jackson's Oxford Journal, (February 27, 1773).

(9)   Oriel College Archives, Bartlemas documents. Oriel Record, (1962), p.10. See also Colin Michie, 'Saint Bartholemew's of Oxford', History Today, 41, (1991), December, p.62.

(10) Will of Samuel Glass, Public Record Office, PROB 11/986 6882

(11) Inventory of Samuel Glass's house. DRO, 72/1/2/ 1. By permission of Devon and Exeter Institution.

(12) Correspondence. DRO, 72/1/2/1. For information on William Wickham's house (34, High Street), see H.E.Salter, Cartulary of the Hospital of St John, I (1914) pp.2712.

(13) Correspondence, DRO, 72/1/2/1.

(14) Ibid.

(15) Ibid.

(16) Ibid.

Appendix to Chapter VI

An uncommon Dropsy from the Want of a Kidney and a Description
of a large Saccus that contain'd the Water.
By Samuel Glass Surgeon at Oxford. Nov 11th, 1746. [Sent to Dr Mead]

Mary Nix who lived at Hampton Poyle a small village in Oxfordshire, had been remarkable all her Life for the preternatural Size of her Belly.

After her Death I had the Curiosity, together with some learned Gentlemen of the University, to inspect her Body. Her Mother was then present and inform'd us that this her Daughter was born Dropsical. That She her Self had been Ill of the same Disease for some Time before and during her Pregnancy, but on the Birth of this Child she was freed from that Disorder.

The Child tho' born Dropsical prov'd otherwise healthy, and notwithstanding the Disease continually increased as She grew up, liv'd to be near twenty three Years of Age. She was a tall well proportion'd Woman except with Regard to the enormous Size of her Belly, and for One of so unwieldy a Bulk, healthy, brisk, and active. Her Appetite was always good, and she was never more than ordinarily thirsty; had no remarkable Difficulty of Breathing, not even when she laid supine,nor did her Thighs or Legs ever swell.

Her Menses which appear'd at the usual Time of Life, continued regular till within eight Months of her Death. The only complaint was now and then a Pain in making Water, and the Quantity she made was commonly about four or five Ounces. Upon the Suppression of her Catamenia, there succeeded a Dyspnoea, Loss of Appetite, Emaciation of the superior Parts, and a Tumefaction of one of her Legs with Ulcerations. These Symptoms gradually increas'd till her Death.

Upon taking the Dimensions of her Body before Dissection we found the Circumference of her Abdomen to be just six Feet four Inches, and from the Xyphoid

Cartilage to the Os Pubis It measur'd four feet and half an Inch. The cutaneous Vessels distributed upon the Abdomen were remarkably large and distended with Blood, and the spurious Ribs were press'd greatly outwards and upwards.

After this general View of the external Parts, We began the Dissection by dividing the Cartilages of the six superior Ribs, and raising the Sternum. The Thorax being laid open, We observ'd that the Diaphragm was forcibly protruded into that Cavity. The Base of the Heart lay under the right Clavicle, and its Apex upon the most convex Part of the Diaphragm which Convexity advanc'd as high up as the third superior Rib. The Lungs were surprizingly small, scarce exceeding in Magnitude those of a new born Child. The right Lobe slightly adher'd to the Pleura, the left was free, and both were in a sound state. Within the Pericardium was found as usual a small quantity of Liquor, but none in the Cavity of the Thorax.

We next perforated the Abdomen in the most convenient depending Part, and evacuated from thence a surprizing Quantity of Water, which was slightly tinged of a Coffee Colour, limpid as urine and not in the least foetid. This Water was carefully measur'd, and found to be not above a Pint less than thirty Gallons Wine Measure, which must weigh according to the common Calculation near 240lb. We afterwards made an Incision along the Linea Alba. The Integuments upon the Epigastric Region were very thin. The Abdominal Muscles much extenuated, and above the Umbilicus the Tunica Cellulosa contain'd no Fat, but from the Navel to the Os Pubis, the Panniculus Adiposus was half an inch thick. Upon dilating the Incision, the large membranous Bag that contain'd the Water presented itself to View, adhering transversly about ten Inches to the anterior Part of the Periosteum. This Adhesion being seperated we had a full View of this wonderful Reservoir, which was of an enormous Size, and had almost occupied the whole Cavity of the Abdomen. In Figure, Colour, Thickness, Number, Magnitude and Distribution of Blood Vessels, it very much resembled the Uterus of a Cow, at the End of Gestation. The whole inside was scabrous, and lookt as if parboil'd, and here and there was observ'd a small Quantity of a Coffee colour'd Sediment. On the left inferior Part was discover'd the Orifice of a Duct, which open'd obliquely into the Cavity of the Saccus, and would easily admit a large Goose Quill. From this Opening the Tube advanc'd about twelve Inches between the Membranes of the Bag, obliquely upward's and toward's the right from where It was inflected downward's, and pass'd between the Duplicature of the Ligamentum latum Uteri, to be inserted into the Bladder of Urine. The Saccus was connected to the Ligamentum Suspensorium Hepatis, to a considerable Part of the Mesocolon, to the Peritoneum on the right Side in two or three different Places, to the same Membrane the whole Length of the Spine, and to the Ligamentum Latum Uteri on the right Side of the Body.

The Liver was sound but less than in a natural state and its convex part adher'd closely to the Diaphragm. The Stomach, Spleen, Omentum, small Intestines, and the upper Part of the Colon were thrust very high up into the left Hypochondrium. The Convolutions of the lower part of the same Intestine were entirely obliterated, and that together with the Rectum formed one continued strait Tube, from the left Hypochondrium down to the Anus.

The left Kidney with its Emulgent Vessels and Ureter were in their natural State and Situation. The Uterus, Tuba Fallopiana, and Ovarium on the same Side had nothing preternatural; but on the right Side the Fallopian Tube and Ovary were dispos'd in a very extraordinary Manner. The Tube by means of the adhesion of the Ligamentum latum Uteri to the Saccus, was extended to three Times its ordinary Length. The Ovary was likewise by the same Cause render'd very preternatural: being no less than five Inches three quarters long, One Inch broad, two tenths of an Inch thick, and two Inches and half distant from the Uterus. The Bladder of Urine was very small, but appear'd to be sound. We then made an accurate Search for the right Kidney, but to our great Surprize found no such Viscus; nor any thing analogous to it, unless the Saccus that contain'd the Water already describ'd, may be esteem'd such: And what seem'd to favour this Opinion, was the Disposition of the Emulgent Vessels on the right Side, which were propagated from the Aorta and Vena Cava to this Saccus, in the same manner as to the Kidney on the opposite Side, and after having run twelve or fourteen Inches between the Membranes of the Bag without any Ramifications, were distributed all over it in the Manner before mention'd.

From the foregoing Account The following Queries are naturally suggested, which I leave to the Determination of the Learned.

Qu: 1. Was not the Saccus originally a mishapen Kidney, and the duct a Ureter?

Qu: 2. Was not the Water contain'd in the Saccus prevented from growing putrid, by being continually drain'd off thro' the Duct into the Bladder of Urine, and by being afresh supplied by the Emulgent Artery, and more being secreted than was evacuated, the Quantity thereby continually increased?

Qu: 3. Was not this the Reason Why the Patient had never any Anasarcous Swellings of her Thighs or Legs, nor any Thirst or other signs of a confirm'd Dropsy?

Qu: 4. Were not the Lungs prevented from growing by the great Diminution of the Cavity of the Thorax, and the pressure they sustain'd from the distended Abdomen; and might not their never having occupied a larger Space than they did at Birth, be the Reason She never labour'd under any Difficulty of Breathing?

Qu: 5. Was not the Bladder of Urine likewise by the Superincumbent Weight, prevented from dilating itself, and that the Reason why the Water was often made, and always in so small a quantity?

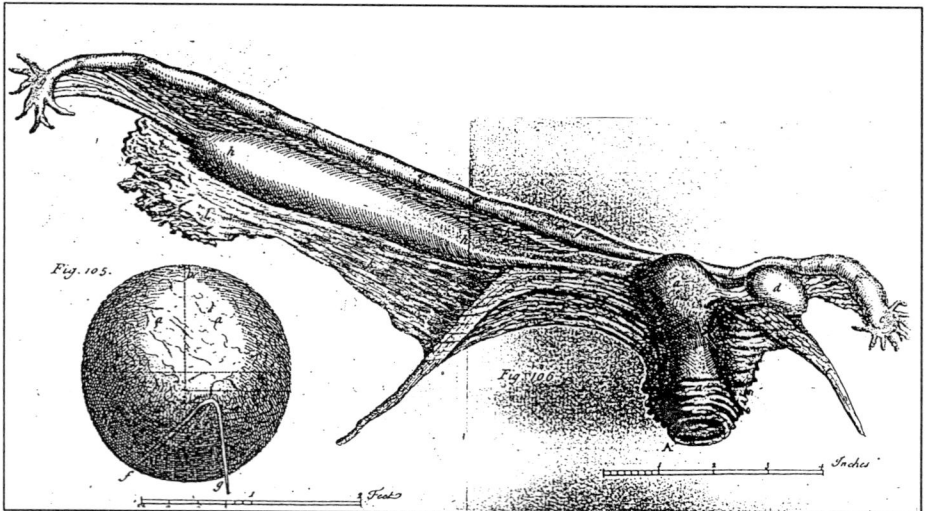

Internal organs taken from Mary Nix at her autopsy.

94

CHAPTER VII
Medical Contemporaries

A physician in a great city seems to be the mere plaything of Fortune; his degree of reputation is, for the most part, totally casual: they that employ him know not his excellence; they that reject him know not his deficiency.

SAMUEL JOHNSON,
Life of Mark Akenside

Biographical details of Thomas Glass's medical contemporaries are somewhat patchy, unsurprisingly. The invaluable *Munk's Roll*[1] provides aid in a small minority, and an even smaller number, like Thomas himself, grace the pages of the *Dictionary of National Biography*.[2] But William Munk's wife was a Devonian, and in 1855 he published a series of articles on Devon Medical Worthies, in the Western Times; J. Delpratt Harris, in 1922, in *The Royal Devon and Exeter Hospital* is invaluable, meticulously combing the minutes of the hospital committee and taking care to verify his facts. Less distant from the eighteenth century, in 1871, Mr. P C. de la Garde, president of the South Western branch of the British Medical Association, fortunately also provided some biographical notes in his presidential address;[3] there are other lay sources, such as the historian, George Oliver.[4]

It was a blow to the surgical staff when John Patch, senior, died at the age of 55, four years after the hospital had opened. His son, likewise named John, was also an original member of the surgical staff, but probably as an assistant to his father, since he was only in his nineteenth year.[5] The elder Patch had learned his profession in Paris, at that time the first school of surgery, and had introduced the operation of lithotomy to the West of England; in France he had been Resident Surgeon to the Pretender's family. John Patch's portrait was painted by his friend, William Gandy, and this may be seen still at the Royal Devon and Exeter Hospital.[6] After his father's death, young John went to Edinburgh to study anatomy, surgery and mathematics. It is said that he had an encyclopaedic mind, a prodigious memory and sound judgment. Furthermore his conversation charmed by its warmth and benevolence. The family lived in Rougemont Castle at Exeter, where he was born; gardening was his recreation and he converted the ditch at the castle 'that foul ravine' into the delightful spot it is today. He befriended the young Opie, who painted the portraits of both him and Thomas Glass in 1783. His reputation as a surgeon extended over a wide area and it was not unusual for him to travel by horseback to Taunton, for example, for a consultation and a fee of five guineas. John died in 1786, at the age of 63.

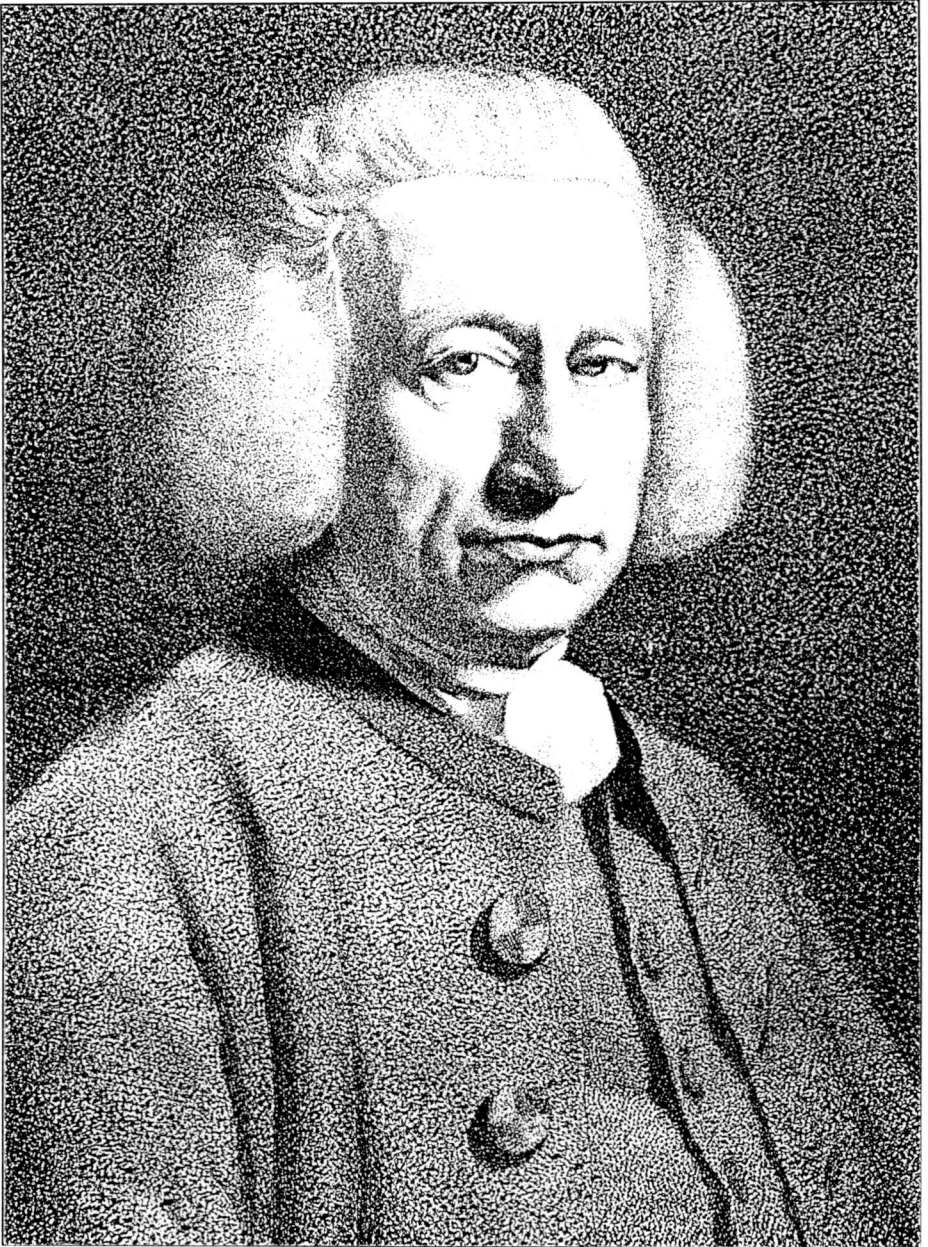

John Patch, junior. Engraving by E.A. Ezekiel from the portrait by Opie.

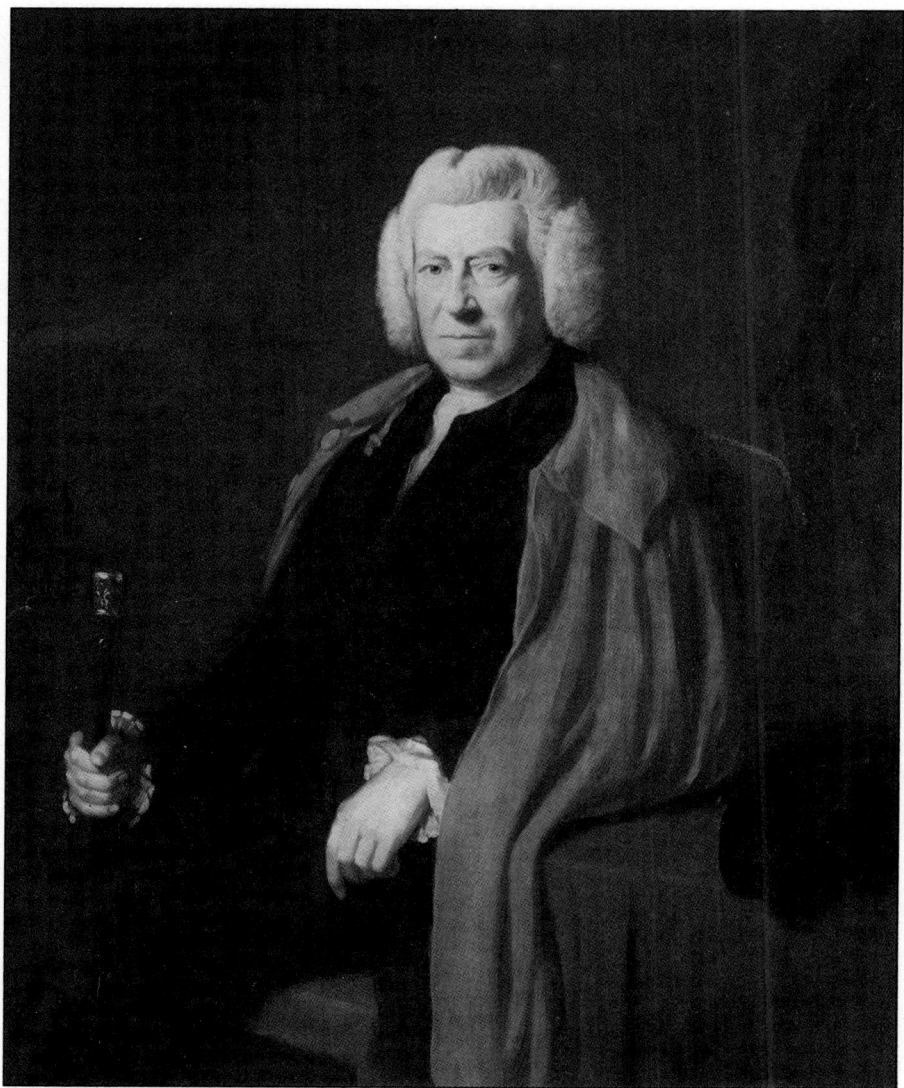

*Thomas Glass by John Opie (1761-1807) circa 1783
(courtesy of Royal Devon & Exeter Healthcare NHS Trust).*

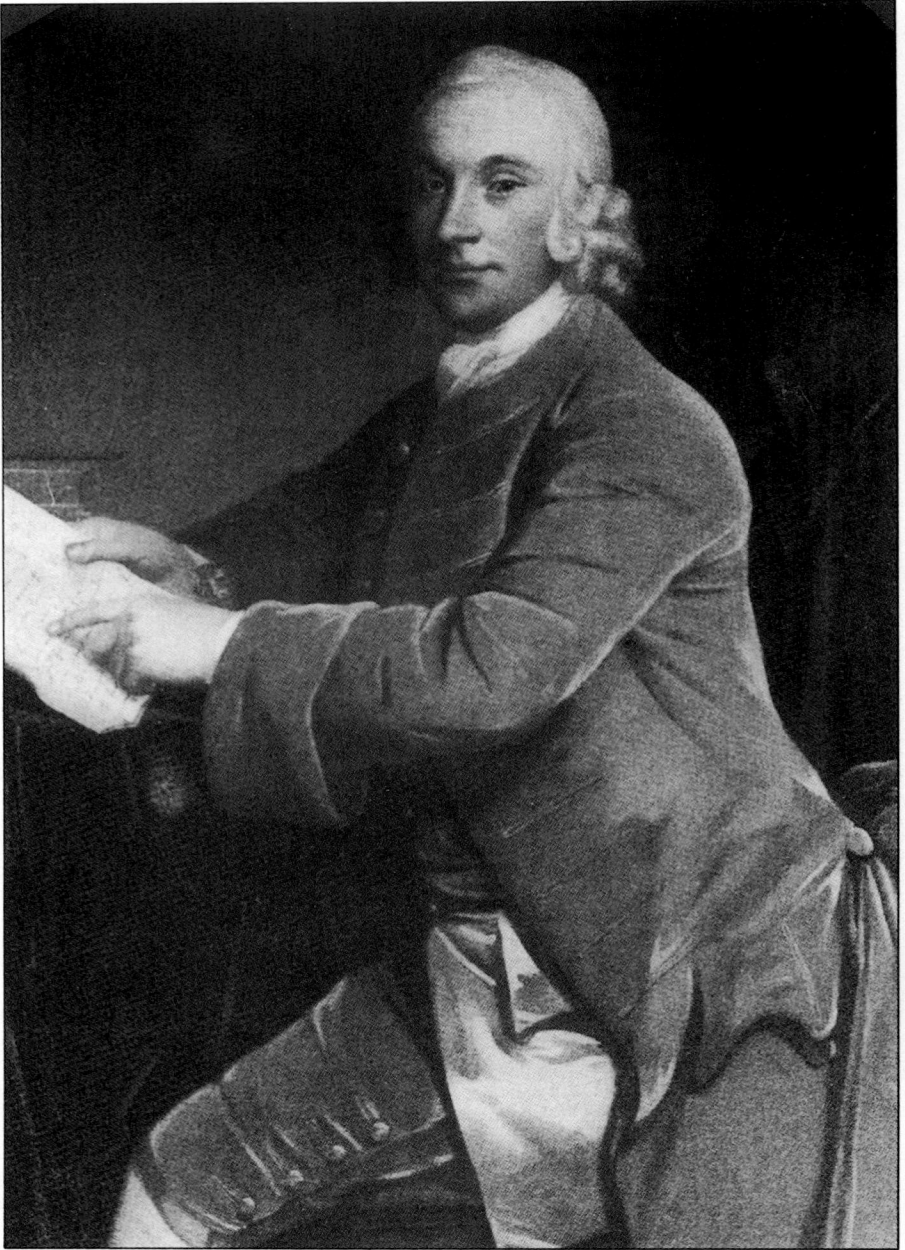

John Andrew by Thomas Hudson (1701-1779)
(courtesy of Royal Devon & Exeter Healthcare NHS Trust).

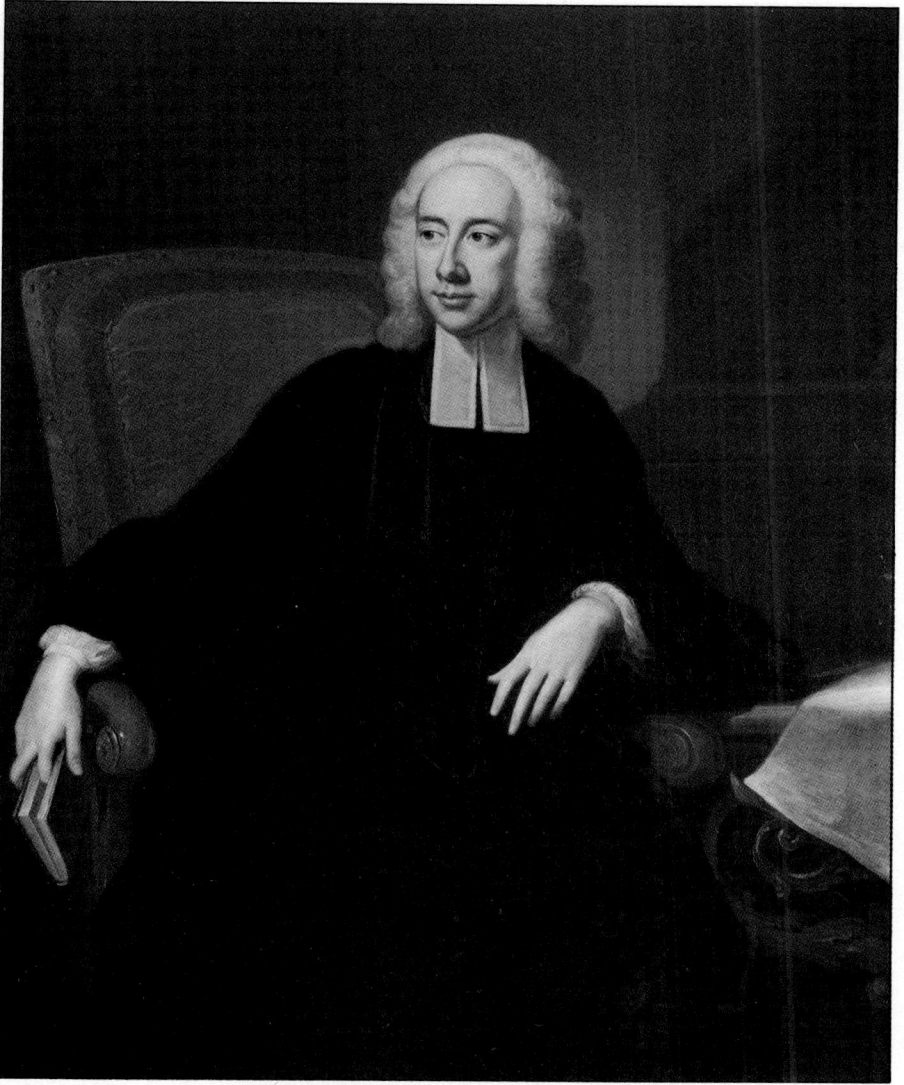

Dean Alured Clarke by James Wills
(courtesy of Royal Devon & Exeter Healthcare NHS Trust).

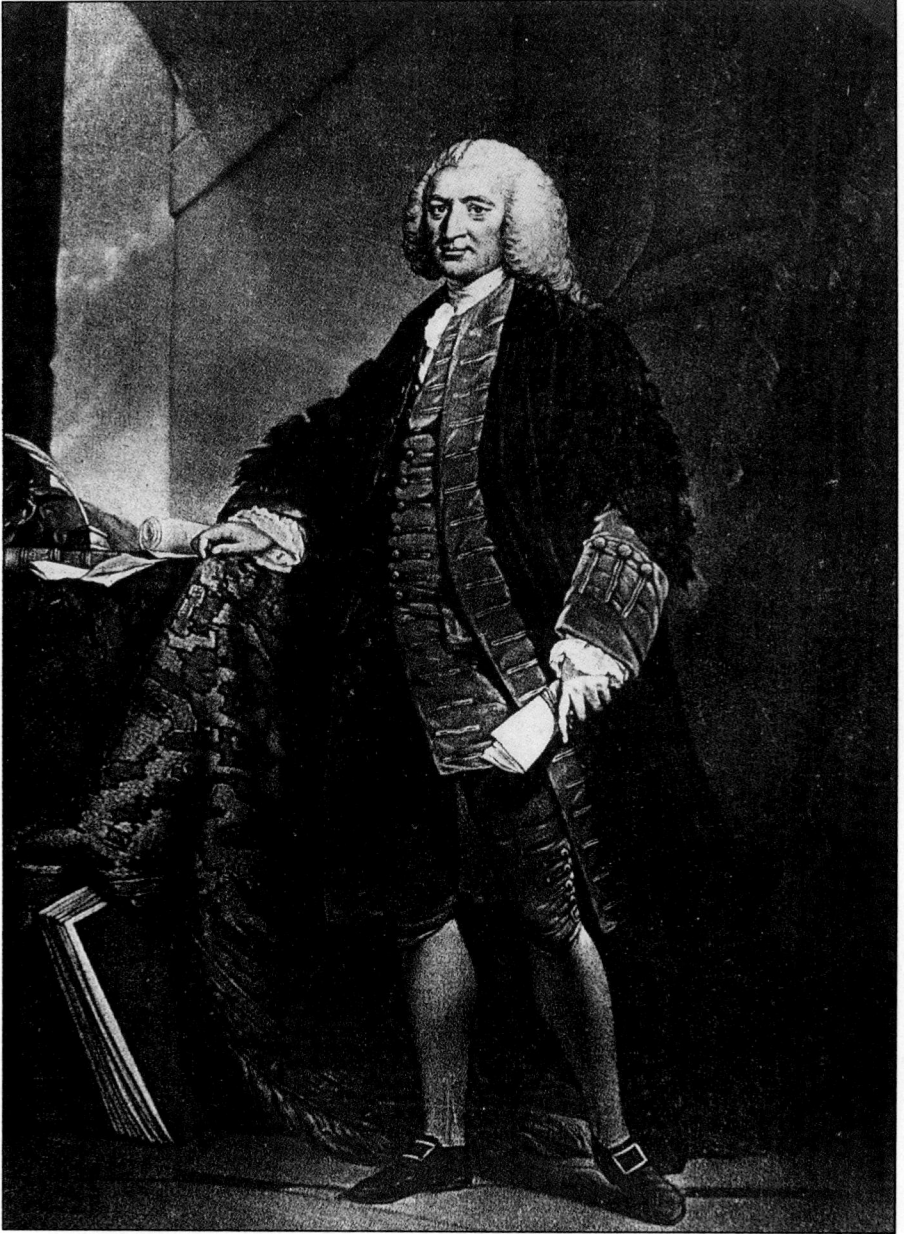

*Benjamin Heath, from the mezzotint engraved by J. Dixon, after the
original painting by R.E. Pine, now in the Guildhall
at Exeter (courtesy Exeter City Council)*

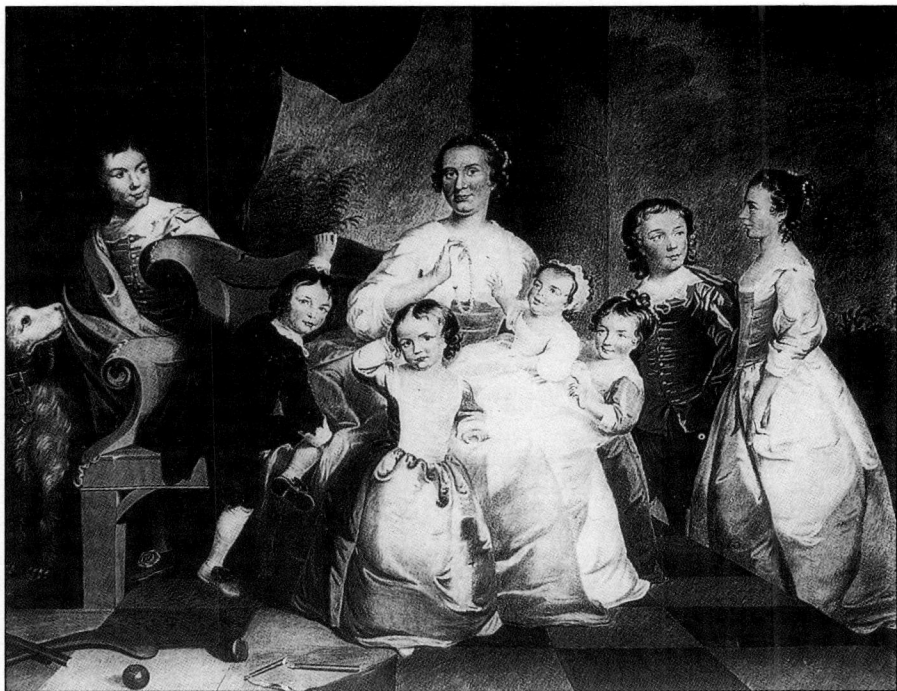

Benjamin Heath's family, from the painting by R.E. Pine.

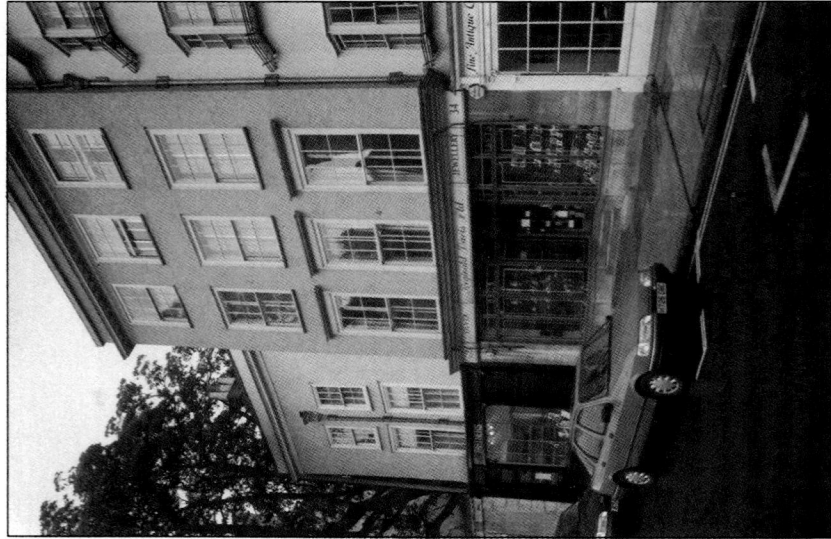

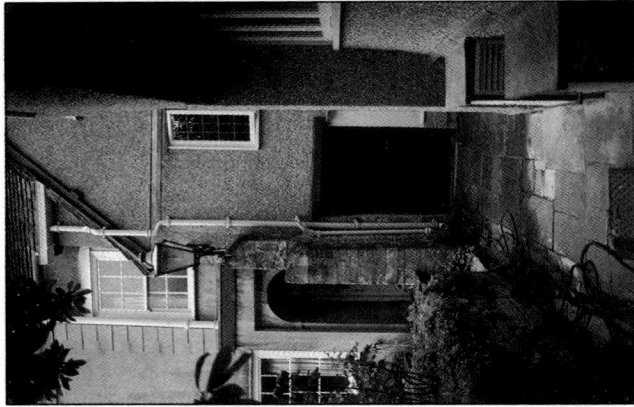

Numbers 33 and 34 High Street, Oxford, the houses occupied by Samuel Glass and William Wickham.

' ...I am sorry to acquaint you that the perpendicular spout between your house and mine, that carries off the water from Mr Glass's house, which is brought down in an angle, made by the projection of my house, is so small, that a very little matter of filth stops it, when the water overflows and spreads and does great damage to your house and mine. My house was so much damaged by the same cause before that the corner post of my house so perished that the three parts in four of it was rotted through and became touchwood.'
William Wickham, 12 May 1775.

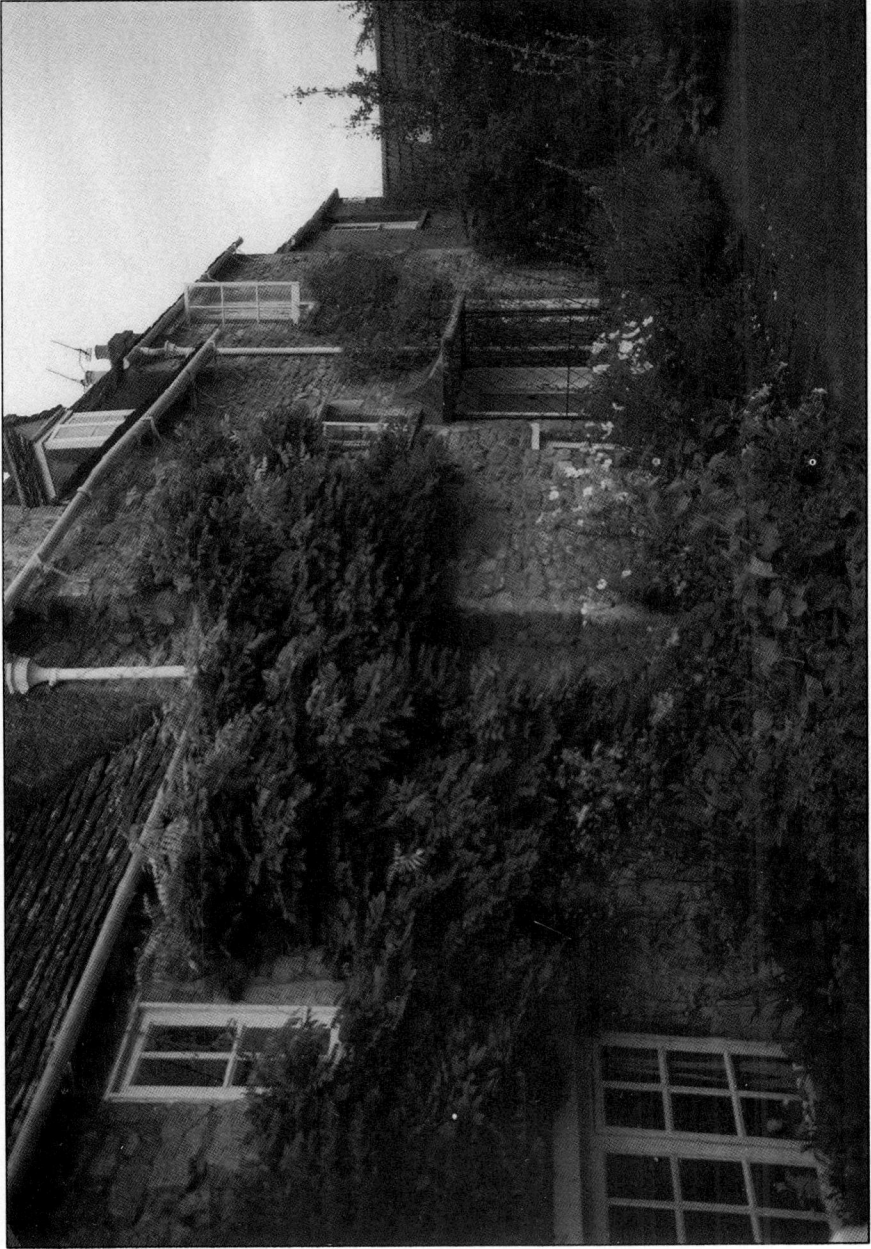

Bartlemas (Bartholemew's farmhouse), 1992.

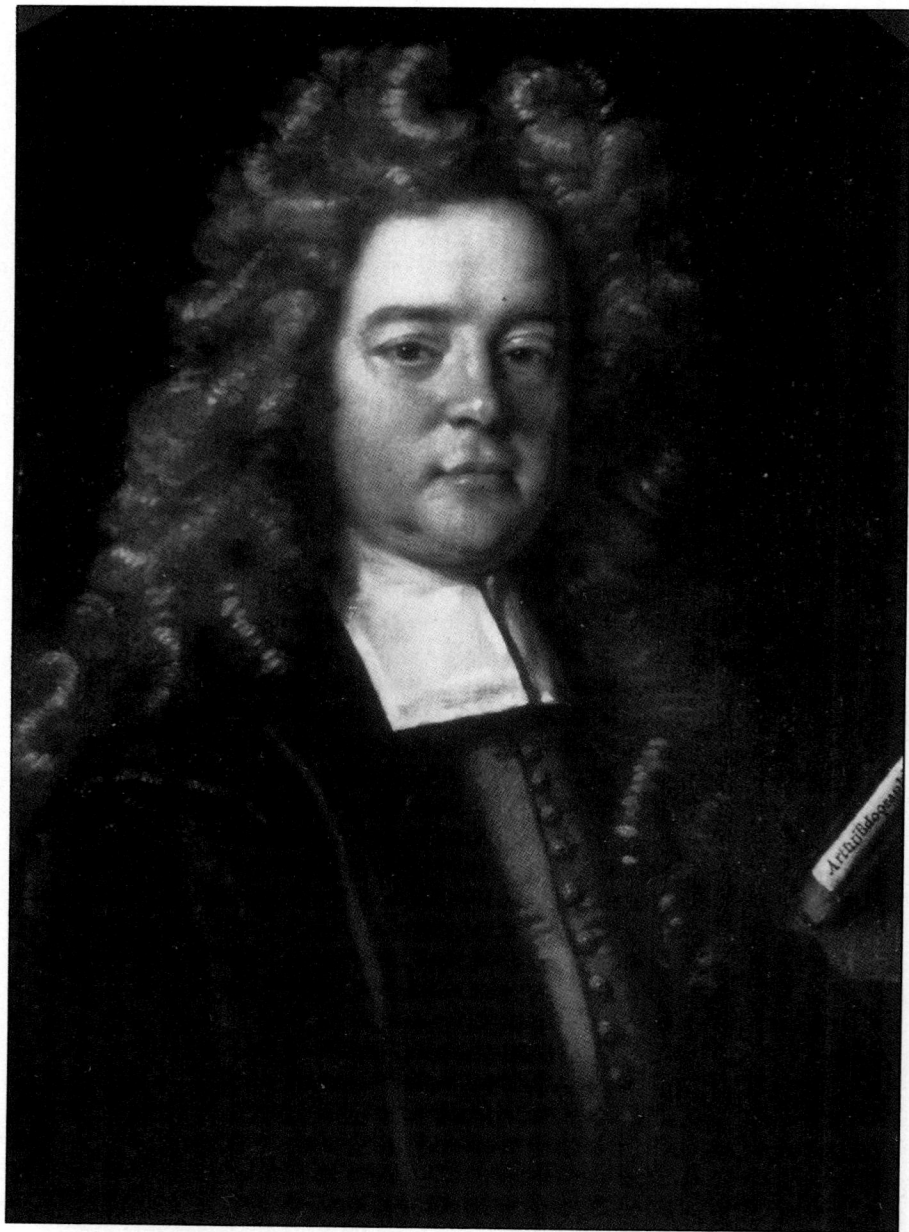

William Musgrave (courtesy Exeter City Council).

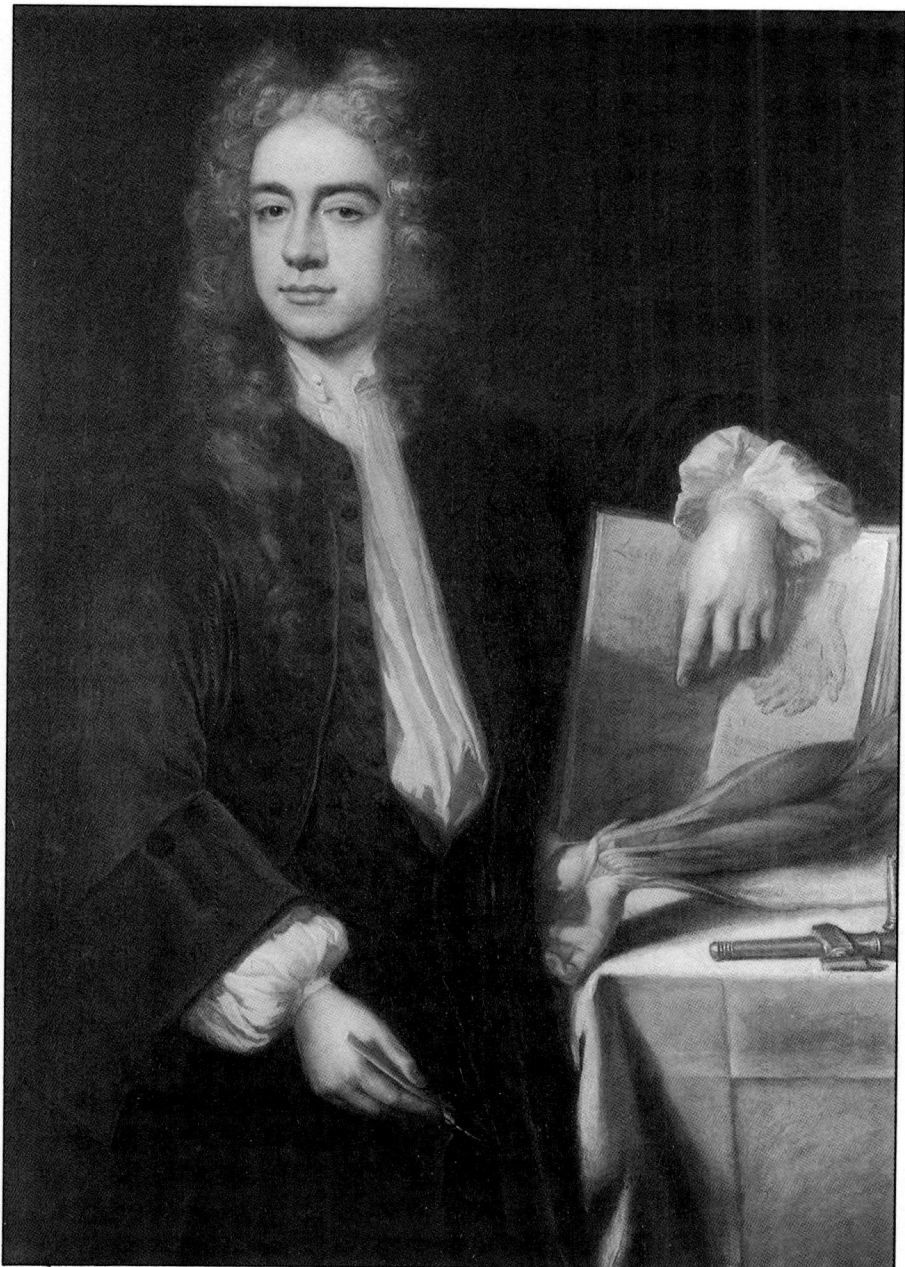

John Patch Senior (1691-1743), by William Gandy.
(courtesy of Royal Devon & Exeter Healthcare NHS Trust).

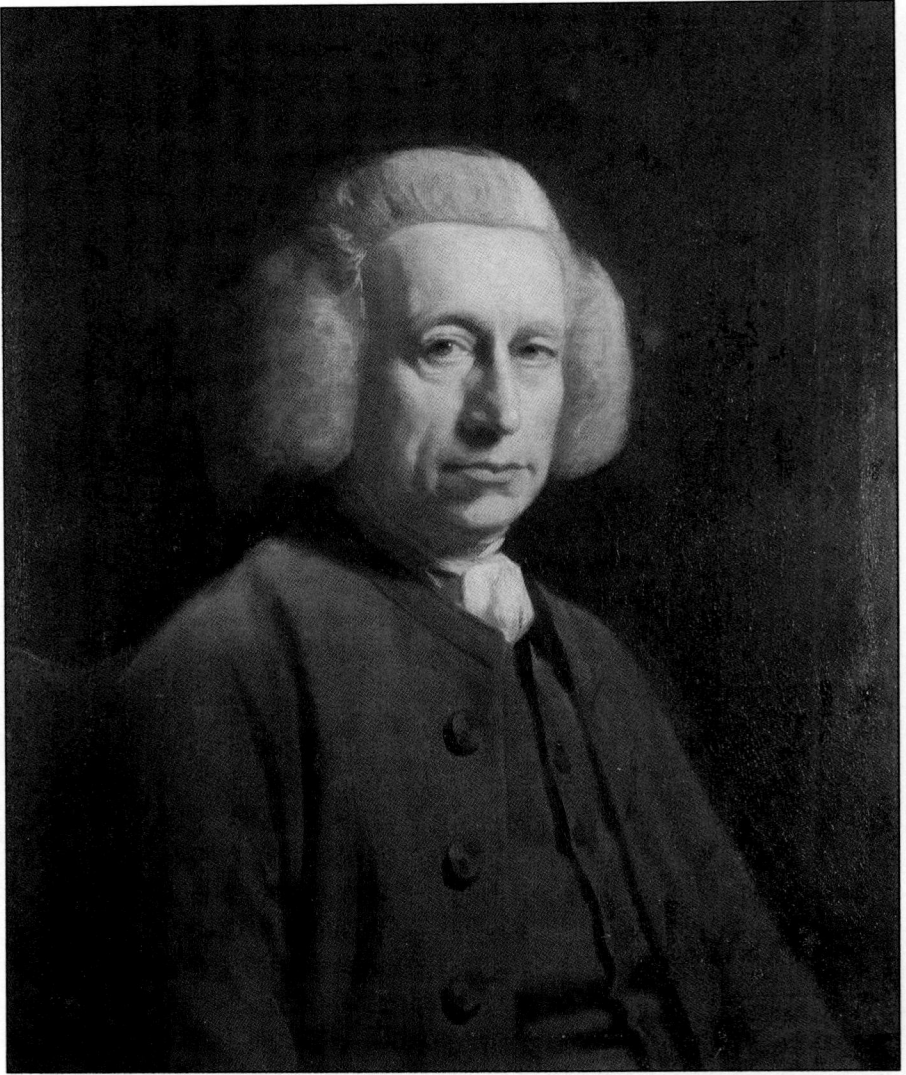

John Patch Junior (1723-1787), by John Opie (1761-1807).
(courtesy of Royal Devon & Exeter Healthcare NHS Trust).

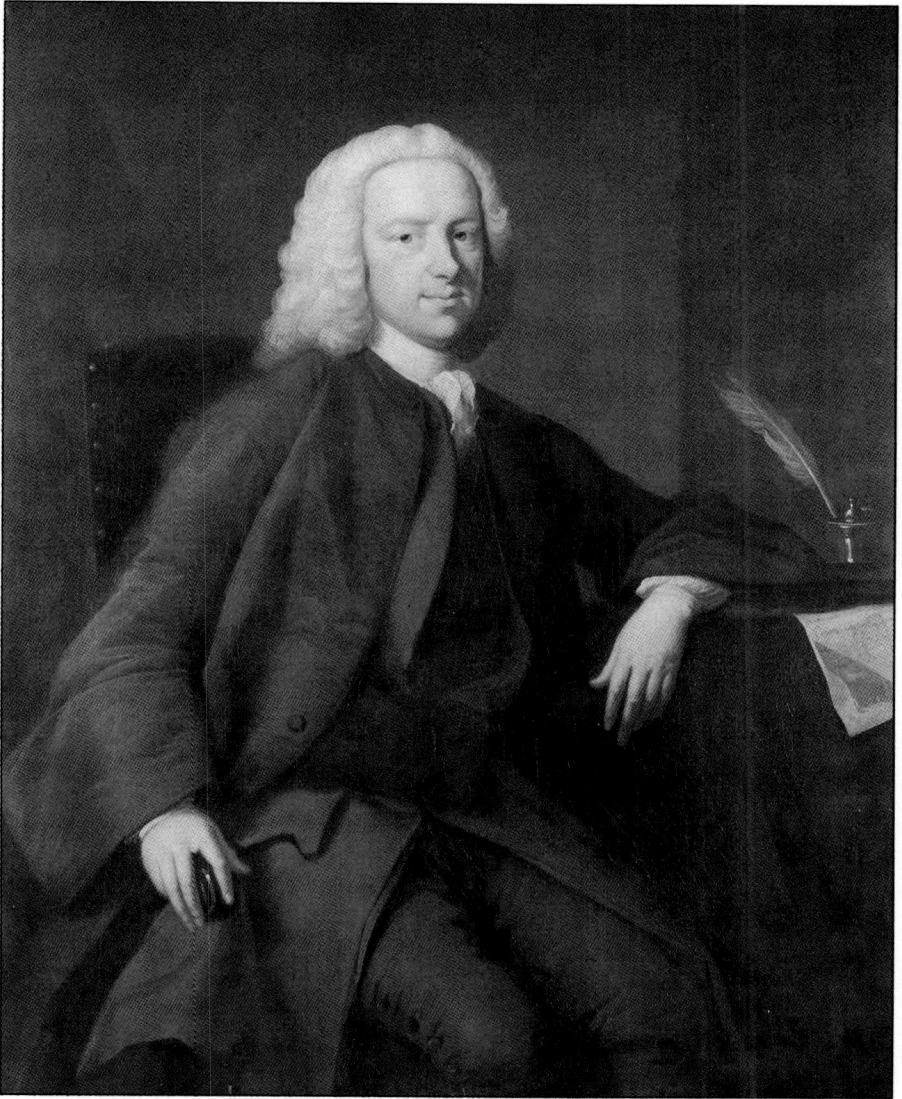

Dr Michael Lee Dicker (1695-1752) by Thomas Hudson (1701-1779)
(courtesy of Royal Devon & Exeter Healthcare NHS Trust).

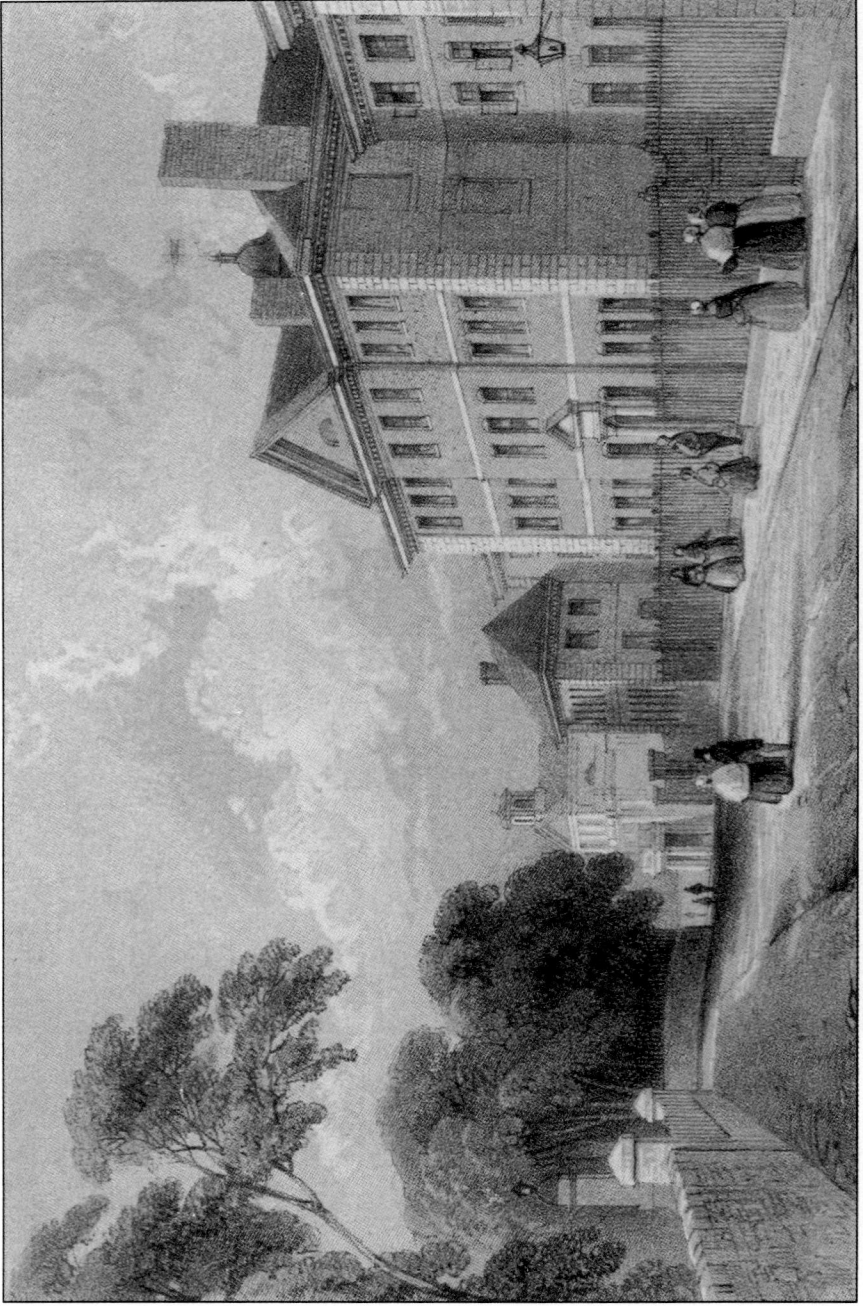

Devon and Exeter Hospital, early 19th century.

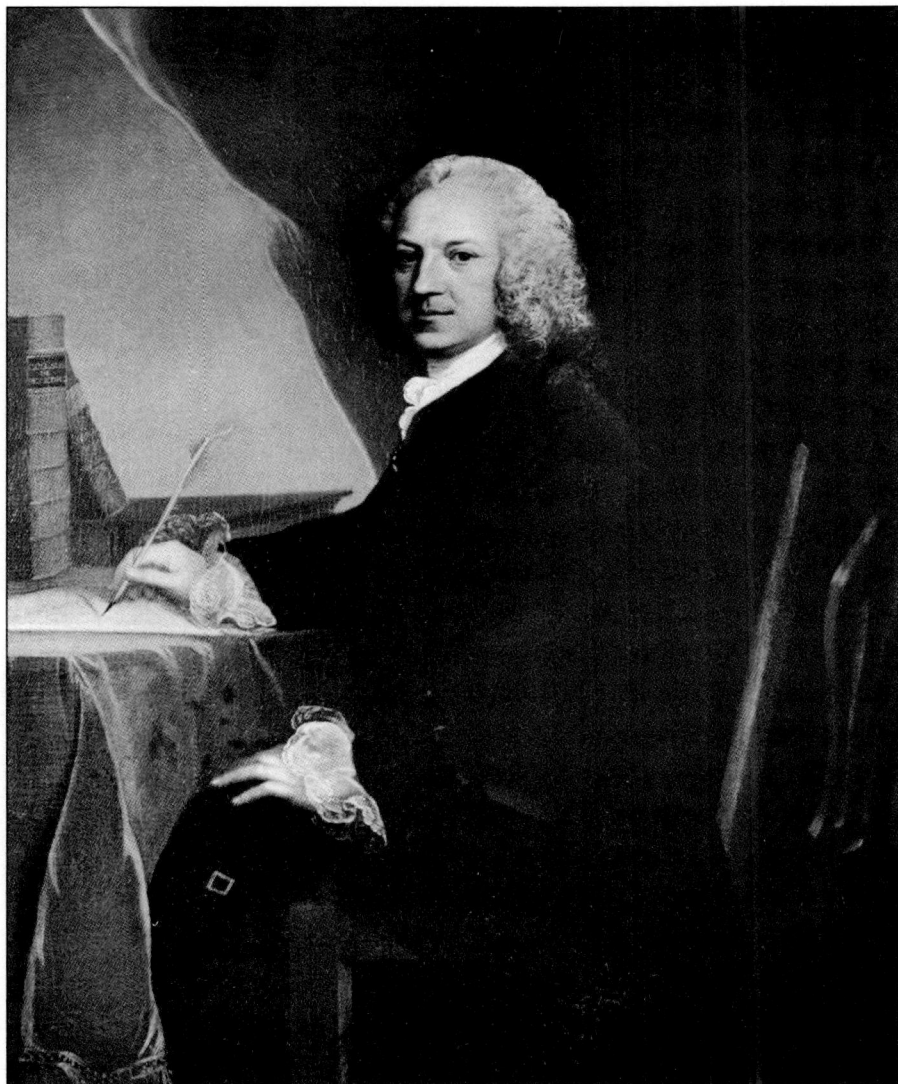

Thomas Glass by Thomas Hudson, circa 1750 (courtesy of Lord Borthwick).

Thomas Glass's Leyden diploma (courtesy of Lord Borthwick).

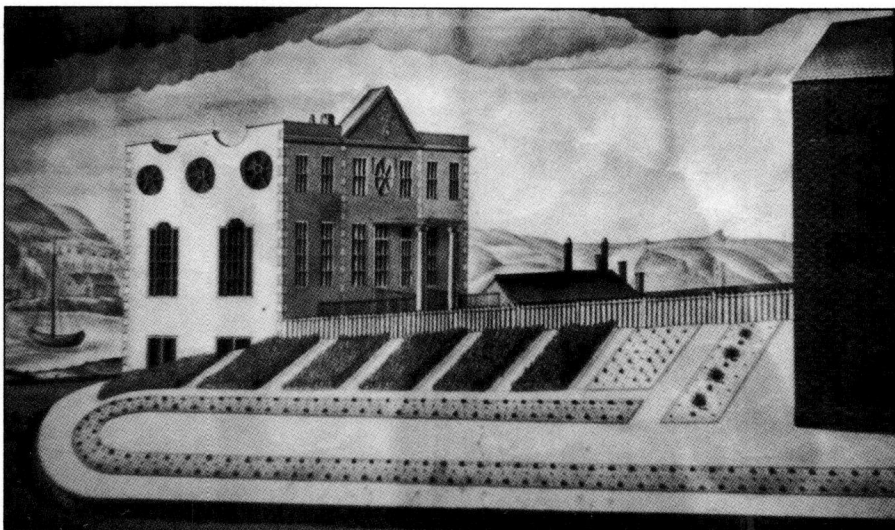

*The Sugar House, Topsham 18th century
by M. Blackamore (courtesy of Mark Mortimer Esq).*

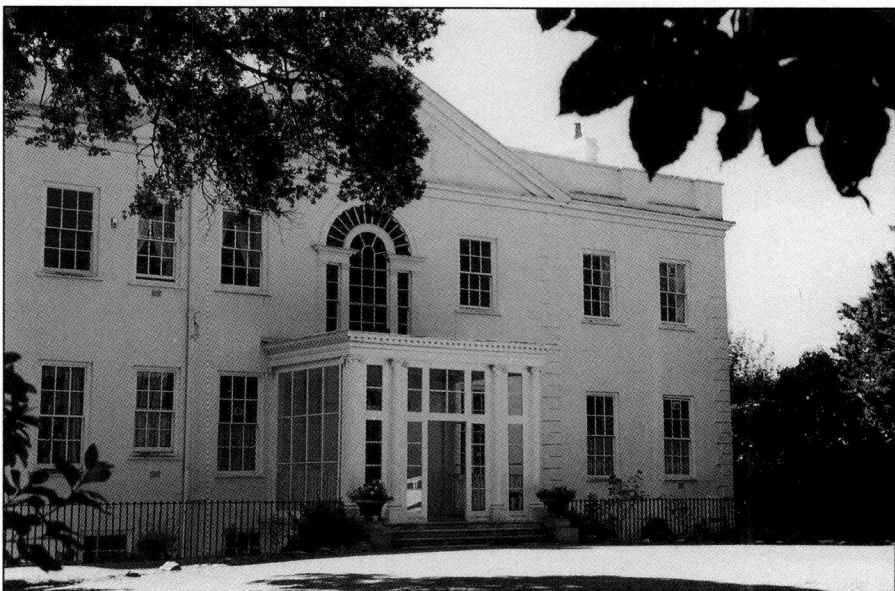

The Sugar House, now called The Retreat, 1991.

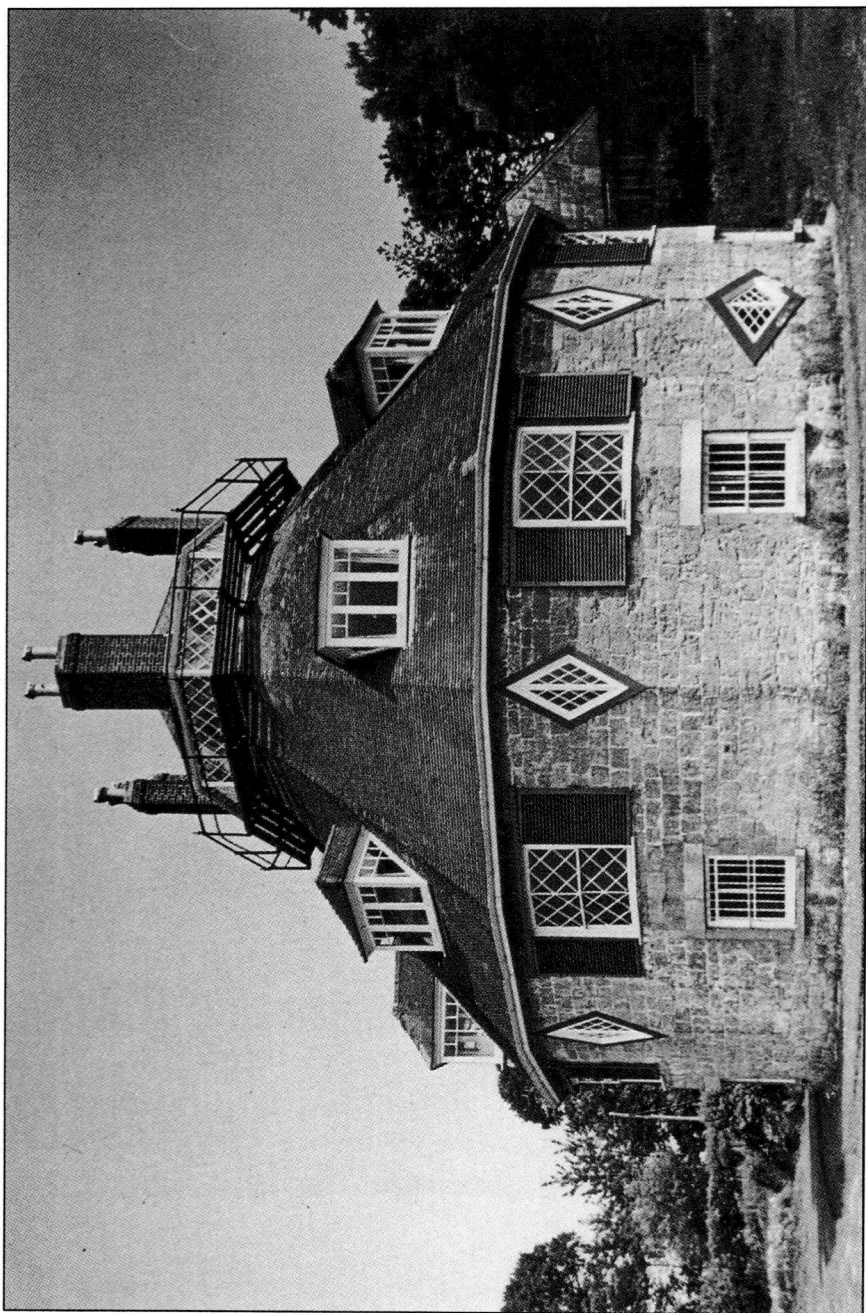

A la Ronde (courtesy of The National Trust).

Hugh Downman, to be mentioned again, wrote a sonnet to John Patch, as he did to many of his friends, which were appended to his Poems to Thespia,[7] love poems addressed to his wife:

> Amid the constant hurry of his time,
> Devoted ever to the public good,
> Shall I to Patch transmit the love-taught rhime?
> On his retirement shall the muse intrude?
> The soul of vigorous, manly sense possest,
> Shall (tho refined) these light productions please?
> Sprung haply from the weak, tho feeling breast?
> Trifling, tho deck'd perchance with grace and ease?
> Yet round the oak the pliant ivy twines,
> His stately trunk not unadorned appears;
> The lofty elm supports the tendrill'd vines,
> Nor less admir'd his branching top he rears.
> So mental intellect, however strong,
> May, undebased, approve the tender song.

Joseph Farington was a friend of the Rev. Gayer Patch, only son of John Patch junior, who gave Farington a thumbnail sketch of his father for whom he had great affection:[8]

> As a surgeon He was at the head of his profession; ... His knowledge was so extensive that from conversing with a child about his 'Tom Thumb' He could go through the depths of Newtonian Philosophy. He was possessed of so much Philanthropy, had so much benevolence ... When he walked through the streets of Exeter every Hat was off to him. The property I possess, said Mr. Patch, I had from my mother; from my Father I should have had nothing. He was too generous for a man who had a view to saving any thing.

The diary continues with a fairly detailed account of a typical day in the life of John Patch, how his nights were so frequently broken in upon by professional calls, followed by a blow by blow record of his customary food and drink, with an emphasis on the latter.

John's brother, James, was also mentioned by Farington. An apothecary surgeon in London, with a good professional reputation, he had 'a severity of natural temperament and was not disposed to make allowances for frailties'. His life ended in 1791 in financial scandal and ruin.

Thomas Patch (1725-1782), another brother of John, was intended for the medical profession in his youth, being apprenticed to an apothecary in Exeter. In the event he became an artist, travelling on the continent with Sir Joshua Reynolds during 1750-1751 and finally settling in Florence, becoming a longtime friend of Sir Horace Mann, the British Ambassador.[9]

A fifth member of this important Exeter medical family was Robert (1750-1813), grandson of the first John, and nephew of the second. The eldest of fourteen children and the son of a clergyman, he was said to be a handsome man and of dignified deportment. He was elected to the hospital staff in 1781; though considered to be a most judicious practioner he was also slow and unhandy as an operator; nevertheless he performed the surgical feat of resecting the humerus at the shoulder in 1803. He was well liked and served the hospital for thirty-two years.[10]

Robert Patch was one of eleven signatories to a letter to Thomas Glass on behalf of the Medical Society of Exeter, on July 4, 1783:

> *Sir,*
>
> *We the members of the Medical Society who have so long been witnesses of the important services you have rendered mankind in your profession at all times, wish to express in the strongest manner the high esteem we have for you, and as one proof of it, we now beg the favour of you to permit your portrait to be taken by an eminent artist, who is soon to be expected in this city.*
>
> *We are fully sensible Sir, that your writings will deliver you down to posterity, but we earnestly wish that the person of him, whose deep learning, nice observation, and sound judgement have done such essential services to his fellow creatures should not be unknown; if you think proper to grant your request we propose to place the portrait in the Board room of the Hospital in which the numbers restored by your means from sickness and from pain, to ease and health, are grateful proofs of your superior abilities.*
>
> *We are with the truest esteem*
>
>
> *Sir, your most humble and obedient servants*
> *Robert Roe Sydenham Peppin William Gater*
> *Thomas Tucker Robert Patch J. Green*
> *Nichs. Arthur Richard Radford*
> *Samuel Luscombe P. Cornish J. Codrington*
>

The reply came from Bartholemew Yard, Exeter, on July 7:

> *Gentlemen,*
>
> *I am very sensible of the singular honour you have conferred upon me, and shall with great pleasure do what you desire.*
>
> *The testimony you have voluntarily and unanimously given me of your esteem, regard, and approbation suggests to me the most pleasing of all reflections, that my life has not been useless to my neighbours; and I account it as my peculiar happiness that I have lived the greatest part of it upon a footing of friendship and have chiefly acted in the business of my profession with such persons as have concurred to erect a monument to the memory of a fellow citizen, because they apprehend he*

may have contributed something towards lessening the sufferings of his
fellow creatures. It is my sincere and earnest wish, that our successors,
both here and elsewhere, may live and act together with as much
harmony and goodwill to each other as we have done.
*   I am, Gentlemen your sincere friend*
*   and obliged humble servant, Thomas Glass.*[11]

Not too many hiccups are recorded in the minute books of the Devon and
Exeter Hospital in its first ten years; by 1752 there were 112 beds occupied by
patients; nursing was provided by eight women, and there was in addition an
apothecary, a matron, and a secretary; below stairs, as it were, a cook, house-
maid, laundry maid and a porter or messenger.

Dr Michael Lee Dicker died in 1752, to whom reference has already been
made. Of all the honorary staff, he had been the most assiduous at attending
meetings, the most frequently placed on sub-committees. His Quakerism
fired his philanthropy, he left money to the hospital, and the Society of
Friends still administer a Dicker Bequest from his relative Samuel Dicker;[12]
corroboration of his humane outlook also springs from another source; a
hardworking German emigré, by the name of Herman Katencamp, lately
employed in the counting-house of John Baring, had in 1744 decided to set up
his own business, when he was brought to the brink of ruin by 'unjust resentment':

his integrity and talents would have been unavailing to save him from
the impending bankruptcy, had not a wealthy and respectable individ-
ual (who had watched his progress for some years. .. and who had from
thence foreseen and predicted his future eminence) at this critical period
stepped forward with offers of assistance, and by the timely loan of
£2000 enjoyed the heartfelt satisfaction of saving a worthy young man
from present ruin and of laying the foundation of his future prosperity
and usefulness. The name of this excellent man, whose character I wish
to hold up as an object of veneration to my Children, was Dicker. He
was a physician and a Quaker, and by his conduct reflected honor both
on his religious and professional practice.[13]

Dicker was awarded his Leyden MD in 1718, his inaugural dissertation being
entitled *de Motibus Ordinatis et Inordinatis Animalium*; the same year he was
made an extra licentiate of the College of Physicians in London.

Quakerism was even reflected in his dwelling in Magdalen Street, where he
built what was known as 'a smart House'. His tenets decreed that a house
should not be highly embellished by ornamentation on the inside and plain
on the outside, where it is exposed to the view of the greater number. In effect
the house was highly decorated on the outside with numerous ornamenta-
tions, dentelles and scrolls giving an unusually smart appearance to it, whilst
the inside was exceedingly plain and more in accordance with Quaker views.

This gave rise to the report that 'Dr Dicker's house is built inside out.'

Michael Dicker's portrait by Hudson, was left to the hospital by the sitter and has survived the intervening centuries.

The name of Dr Richard Mead (1673-1754), that ornament of eighteenth century medicine in London, recurs here and there, but only on the fringe of the life of Exeter. As a fellow bibliophile, he was a close friend of Benjamin Heath and it was to him that the latter dedicated his unpublished Notes on Catullus:

Viro amplissimo atque Ornatissimo
Omni Eruditionis genere praestantissimo,
Omnium in unoquoque genere Eruditorum Maecenati eximio,
Tantumque non unico,
Ricardo Mead, M.D.,
Hunc qualemcunque Libellum
Ea, qua par est, veneratione reverentia inscribit,
Privatum hoc grati animi Testimoniuum,
Ob publica sua in rem literariam merita,
Quibus omnes Literarum Cultores sibi in aeternum devinxit,
Exstare cupiens
Dexiades Ericius[14]

The quaint *nom de plume* used by Benjamin Heath - *Dexiades Ericius* -may be rendered literally as 'right-handed hedgehog' and is full of classical allusion. The biblical Jacob had dubbed his youngest son Benjamin - the son of his right hand; ericius is a punning reference to the Latin ericaeus, of heath or ling, or the Greek εριкαευς, heathery. Thomas Glass and Mead were also acquainted, as witness this letter inside a presentation copy of Mead's *Concerning the Influence of the Sun and Moon upon Human Bodies:*

Ormond Street, August 7th, 1746.

Dear Sir,
I have ordered my bookseller to send you a copy of the next edition of my book de Imperio Solis etc, which though a Triffle I beg your acceptance of, as a mark of the great respect and esteem with which I am
Sir,
Your most obedient humble servant
R.H.Mead

Mead also presented Glass with a copy of his *Discourse on the Smallpox*.[15]

There are other books amongst those bequeathed by Thomas Glass, which had been dedicated specifically to him, indicating the respect of his contemporaries; Nicholas May, for instance, a surgeon from Plymouth, mentioned in chapter three. Another was a Leyden inaugural dissertation concerning smallpox and measles, by Edward Spry, in 1768. This was dedicated to a veritable army of British and continental medical worthies, but especially and in the most fulsome terms to the 'most eminent, most celebrated and most amicable doctors of medicine Huxham, Andrew and Glass'. Spry, needless to say, came from the West Country.

Two more medical names, in this post-Augustan city of Exeter, glimmer through the haze of the intervening centuries; they are those of Musgrave and Downman.

Samuel Musgrave (1732-1780) is accorded five pages in Munk's Roll, but it is the tragic account of an exceptionally gifted classical scholar, whose career swerved violently from the straight path in a bizarre and capricious fashion, terminating in an early death in abject poverty.

He was the great-nephew of William Musgrave (1655-1721), but not as some have said his grandson.[16] William was a distinguished Exeter physician and FRS, who published two medical classics: *De Arthritide Symptomatica* and *De Arthritide Anomala*. The first of these records the history of another Exeter physician, Malachi Thruston F.R.S (1629-1701), not named but identifiable, who was William's patient, and who ended his life in madness[17]. *De Arthritide Primigenia et Regulari* was found in manuscript at his death and subsequently published at Oxford in 1726, and by Samuel in 1776. He was a noted antiquary and an authority on the Roman occupation of Britain, hence his large four-volume work *Antiquitates Brittano-Belgicae* (1711, 1716, 1719, 1720). William was second secretary of the Royal Society for some years, contributing to and editing the Philosophical Transactions, from No. 167 to No. 178.

When John Patch senior had his portrait painted by Gandy in 1717, William wrote a dedicatory inscription to the sitter, which for many years was tucked between the picture and the frame; it reflects with affectionate humour the essence of the writer as much as of the subject.[18]

Samuel was born at Washfield, in Devon, and educated at the grammar school of Barnstaple, then at Corpus Christi college, Oxford, as a scholar. Being elected to a Radcliffe travelling fellowship in 1756, he went abroad, dividing his time between Holland and France and graduating MD at Leyden in 1763. Before this, in 1760, the young man sent to the press, in London, *Some Remarks on Dr Boerhaave's Theory of the Attrition of the Blood in the Lungs*, and in 1762 he published at Leyden *Exercitationes duae in Euripidem*. It was perhaps in keeping with his temperament, forthright and questioning, that he should choose a subject for his MD dissertation calculated to be at variance with established views, a learned essay in defence of empirical medicine.[19] Empiricism was certainly regarded with universal disfavour, on a par with quackery.

When in Paris, on leaving Leyden, he was elected a corresponding member of the Royal Academy of Inscriptions and Belles Lettres. He dallied in France until the expiry of his Radcliffe fellowship, and it seems possible that his questing mind led him to dabble in politics, thus sowing the seed of his ultimate destruction. He returned to Exeter with the seed germinating in his heart, and was elected physician to the Devon and Exeter hospital on July 24, 1766.

It is said that Samuel found the Exeter ground fully occupied by doctors Andrew and Glass, but whether through impatience or impulsiveness, he soon sought new pastures. The minutes of the hospital committee record that in August, 1768, he had recommended an apparatus for a poor girl who was incapacitated, which the committee granted. The following month they received a laconic letter from Plymouth, acquainting them that he had settled there and could no longer look after his patients in the hospital.

Then followed the political hand grenade, tossed by Samuel into the arena the following year, when he published *An Address to the Gentlemen, Clergy, and Freeholders of the County of Devon.*[20] During his residence in Paris in 1764, he said, he had received trustworthy information that an overture had in that year been made to certain influential members of Parliament, in the name of the Chevalier d'Eon, importing that he, the Chevalier was ready to impeach three persons, two of whom were peers of the realm and privy councillors, of selling the then recent peace to the French Government.[21]

On his return to England, Samuel obtained an interview with Lord Halifax, then Secretary of State, when he communicated the information he had received, urging him to question the Chevalier. His lordship was described as polite but evasive and requested documentary evidence; Samuel thereupon submitted copies of four letters to and from Lord Hertford, bearing on the subject. Halifax declined to take any action, as did the Speaker of the House of Commons, Samuel's next port of call. Here the matter rested for a while, though subsequent to his interview with Lord Halifax, Samuel had been informed by Mr Fitzherbert that an approach had been made to the Chevalier d'Eon to purchase the papers from him.

It would seem that Musgrave acted from the highest motives, in the mould of Wilkes; it may have been delusion or he may have been on the brink of uncovering political skulduggery of the most sensitive kind. Why else risk professional ruin at Plymouth where prospects were good and there was a medical vaccuum, following the death in 1768 of John Huxham? Indeed he claimed credit for pure patriotism and a desire to visit with befitting punishment those who, high in the councils of this country, had proved traitors to its interests. The address opened a Pandora's box of pamphlets, and an immediate response from the Chevalier d'Eon, who repudiated all knowledge of Dr Musgrave, and emphatically denied everything that had been advanced concerning himself. A full hearing in the House of Commons pronounced the assertions to be frivolous and unworthy of credit.

These matters were widely reported in the press, in particular the *Gentleman's Magazine* and the *Oxford Magazine*, the latter printing several cartoons.[22] One of these depicts Dr Musgrave prescribing for Britannia 'who is in a deep Consumption,' his words to her are 'be comforted, you may yet revive'. In another the Chevalier d'Eon is seen vomiting on Lord Bute and others, following an emetic administered by Samuel, who is strategically placed behind him with a gigantic enema syringe to be used if necessary. The

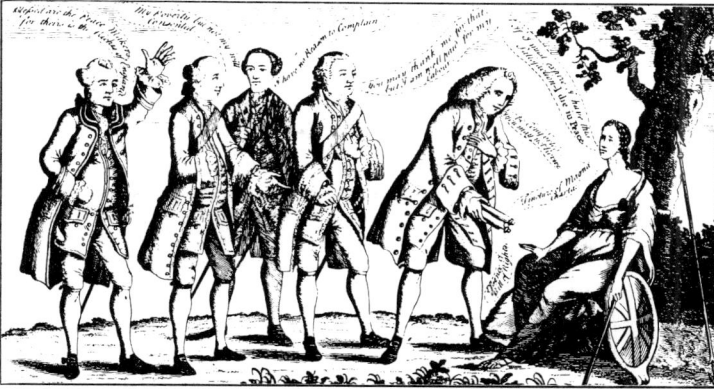

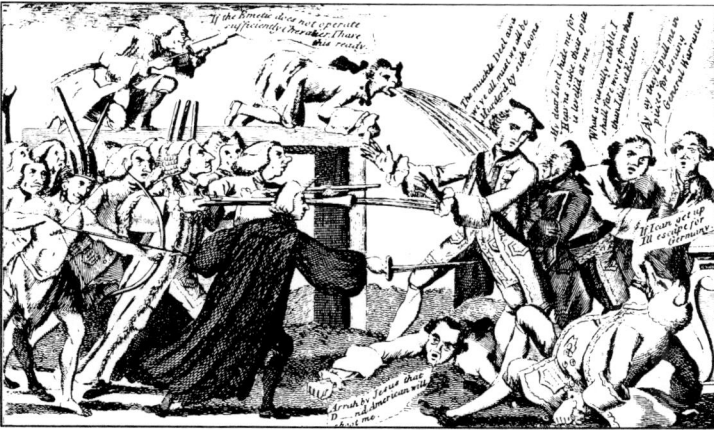

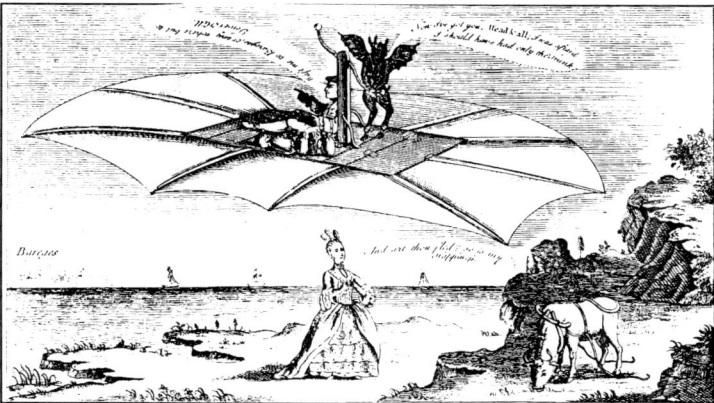

Three cartoons from the Oxford Magazine, *1769, depicting Samuel Musgrave, the Chevalier d'Eon, Lord Bute, and others (by permission of Centre for Oxfordshire Studies, Central Library, Oxford).*

principal villains in Samuel's eyes, apart from the Chevalier, were the Marquis of Bute, Lord Hertford and the Duke of Bedford; the latter became very unpopular in Exeter, partly on this account, but also because he had been associated with the hated cider tax, and in 1769 he received rough treatment from the Exeter mob, from whom he had to beat a hasty retreat.[23]

This was all too much for the people of Plymouth, and after a fruitless interval Samuel determined to try his luck in London. Here he tried to earn his living by his pen, some of his writing was political, but after 1772 he concentrated on medical matters and the classics. Acknowledged as an authority on Euripedes, his manuscript notes for his dissertations on this author were considered so valuable that Oxford University purchased them for £200.

In 1775 he took his degree of Doctor of Medicine at Oxford, and in 1777 was elected a Fellow of the College of Physicians. He gave the Gulstonian Lectures at the College in 1779.

He was known to Samuel Johnson and is referred to by Boswell at a dinner which they attended, the learned Dr Musgrave's contribution to the conversation is described.[24] There is also an interesting suggestion that Samuel might have been that enigmatic figure Junius, the *nom de plume* of the writer of a series of telling letters to the *Public Advertiser*, so critical of the government of George III, from January 1769, to January 1772.[25]

As a bizarre envoi to this bizarre tale, it seems that when the Chevalier d'Eon died, at the age of 86, in 1810, it was confirmed that, as had been long suspected, he could more properly have been described as Chevalière, since he was in reality a woman.[26]

Samuel's last desperate efforts to obtain notice and practice met with failure, his circumstances became more and more embarrassed, and he died at his lodgings on July 5, 1780, aged 47.

Hugh Downman (1740-1809) was educated at Exeter Grammar School, went thence to Balliol and was ordained in Exeter Cathedral in 1763. Finding his clerical prospects to be small, and already having become attached to Dr Andrew's second daughter, Frances, he took himself to Edinburgh to study medicine, returning to Exeter in 1770 to practise and to marry Frances.

Hugh was a poet and, almost certainly, a consumptive. His best known poem was *Infancy, or the Management of Children*. It seems odd in these days that a very long didactic poem, like this, could ever become a paediatric best-seller, and yet it went into nine editions and is full of good advice. The poem is written in Miltonic blank verse, in a style that combines flowery classicism, somewhat incongruously, with medical phraseology:

> *Angina, aphthous sores, Eruptions dire,*
> *Pertussis fierce, and squalid Atrophy.*

As Miss J.M.S.Tomkins commented:

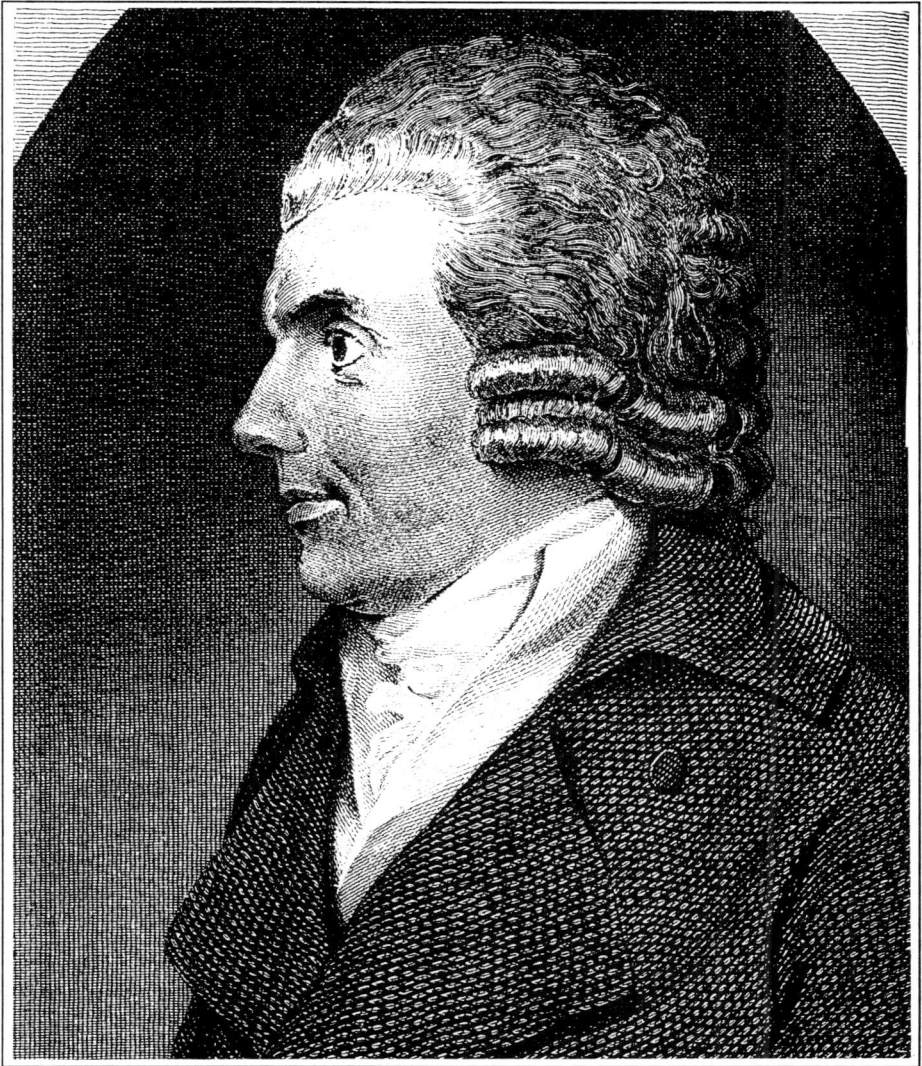

Hugh Downman, from a painting by John Downman. Engraved by John Fittler.

his grand foe is ancient superstition, too often incarnated in the figure of the midwife. On the threshold of the poem she stands, a sinister figure, preparing for the newborn child the poisonous drench that custom sanctified and advancing science condemned.[27]

He is described as having a 'chronic complaint' and certainly his life was fractured by ill health; this led him to resign from the hospital in 1778, returning to the staff in 1784; during his long indisposition he lived 'close on the verge of want'. He finally retired from the hospital in 1802 and from medical practice in 1805. A biographical Memoir appears in the *Gentleman's Magazine*,[28] in which it is said:

> *In form, Dr Downman, in the earlier periods of his life, was strong and athletic, nor till his health was undermined by indulgence and inactivity, did he appear an invalid. Notwithstanding the influence of these destructive habits, his constitution appeared firm and vigorous; and he struggled against disease, with a force little to be expected from his appearance. He seemed to have been built for a life much longer than that which he enjoyed, or perhaps more properly, if the whole be considered, he endured.*

At one point in his poem *Infancy* he appears to refer to his own health in a moment of introspection:

> *Can I then hope, whom sickness long hath drench'd*
> *In her Lethean dews, with feeble limbs,*
> *And wan complection, from her hands to bear*
> *Those gifts, which unpossest, my lays must creep*
> *Dully monotonous, nor touch the heart,*
> *Nor win th' approving mind? Yes, witness Thou!*
> *Witness my Friend! Who know'st the human frame,*
> *Each drug of cordial, each of healing power,*
> *To me in vain administer', what toil*
> *I must experience now, The Nymph to trace*
> *Through her meand'ring walks! what partial chance*
> *Should she my languid homage not disdain!*[29]

A fellow sufferer would certainly recognize being 'drench'd in her Lethean dews'.

There are generous references to his Edinburgh teachers, Cullen, Gregory, Monro, and Black; Glass is mentioned in the same breath as Huxham, Boerhaave, and Sydenham:

> *While Glass with evening brightness still adorns*
> *The Western Sky, and proves not yet extinct*
> *The true, the genuine Hippocratic beams.*[30]

This surely was an indication of the pedestal on which he had placed his former senior colleague, counter to Parr, who incidently was never accorded the compliment of a Downman verse.

Among the many sonnets addressed to local figures, are some to those already mentioned elsewhere, such as Archdeacon Sleech; some rather pedestrian, others with great tenderness and delicacy of touch, such as that to Mrs Andrew, his mother-in-law.[31] These, however, are appended to the many love poems addressed to his wife, Frances (alias Thespia).

In 1792 the Literary Society was established at Exeter, which had initially nine, later twelve, members;[32] Hugh Downman was the founder and first president, and among its number were Richard Polwhele, John Sheldon, the Rev. Richard Hole, and Bartholemew Parr. Isaac d'Israeli, father of Benjamin, spent three years in Exeter at about this time and was a friend and patient of Downman; he also was a member.[33]

The seaside town of Dawlish has much to thank Hugh Downman for, as it was he who, in *Infancy*, first promoted it as a desirable and salubrious watering place.

Notes

(1)   William Munk, *The Roll of the Royal College of Physicians of London*, (London, 1878).

(2)   William and Samuel Musgrave, Richard Mead, and Hugh Downman are mentioned.

(3)   Philip Chilwell de la Garde, F.R.C.S., (1797-1871), was senior surgeon of the Devon and Exeter Hospital and Exeter Eye Infirmary. Copies of the address were printed, (Exeter, 1871); one is held at the Postgraduate Medical Centre at the Royal Devon and Exeter Hospital.

(4)   'Curiosus' (Revd. George Oliver), 'Biographies of Eminent Exonians', mid 19th C newspaper cuttings (probably *Western Times*), located at the Devon and Exeter Institution. (Stones Scrapbooks)

(5)   J. Delpratt Harris, *The Royal Devon and Exeter Hospital*, (Exeter, 1922), p. 63.

(6)   Ibid, p. 26.

(7)   Hugh Downman, *Poems to Thespia*, (Exeter, 1792), p. 144.

(8)   *The Diary of Joseph Farington*, (London,1926), Vol. VI, p. 184.

(9)   Ibid, p.181 and *DNB*.

(10) P.C. de la Garde, op.cit., p.9.

(11) J. Delpratt Harris, op.cit., p.50.

(12) Devon and Cornwall Quarterly Meeting of the Society of Friends, *Trust Property within the County of Devon*, (London,1899), p. 11.

(13) Anna W. Merivale, *Family Memorials*, (Exeter, 1884), pp. 67,68.

(14) The dedication to Mead appears in Sir William R. Drake, *Heathiana*, (London, 1881), p. 10.

(15) Both these books are in the medical section of Exeter Cathedral Library.

(16) P.C. de la Garde, op.cit., p.7, is clearly incorrect in stating that William was Samuel's grandfather, from their respective entries in *DNB*. See also Devon and Cornwall Notes and Queries, XII, p.264.

(17) *De arthritide symptomatica...*, (London, 1703), pp 83-87.

(18) The portrait shows Patch demonstrating the dissection of an arm. The inscription, written in Latin by William Musgrave in 1717, was in his own handwriting, according to J. Delpratt Harris; pointing out that it was an exordium to a picture and not an obituary, he gives the following translation

Here you have a man
Proved as an anatomist
Skilful as a surgeon
  As the latter prosperity is pointed out by the mouth
  As the former by the hand of the dead.
Rejoice patrons of medicine
Be pleased lovers of pictures
Gandy painted John Patch
Who would give life to a giver of life.
  Reader
  What you look at trust as a memorial of friendship.

See Delpratt Harris, op.cit. p.26. The original has been lost.
(19) *Dissertatio Medica inauguralis sive Apologia pro Medicina Empirica*, Leyden, 1763.
(20) *Exeter Flying Post*, August 12, 1769.
(21) The Peace of Paris terminated the Seven Years War.
(22) *Gentleman' Magazine*, November, 1769, passim; *Oxford Magazine*, 1769, passim.
(23) Robert Newton, *Eighteenth Century Exeter*, (Exeter, 1984), p.78.
(24) James Boswell, *The Life of Samuel Johnson*, (London, 1901), Vol III, pp 2, 3.
(25) This suggestion was made by de la Garde, op. cit., p.8, on the grounds that the style of the two writers was very similar, and that they were both politically active between the same dates, i.e. January 21st, 1769, and January 21st, 1772. More conventional opinion seems to favour Sir Philip Francis, Edmund Burke, or Tom Paine as the real Junius.
(26) See Farington, op.cit., p.62.
(27) J.M.S.Tomkins, 'The Didactic Lyre', in *The Polite Marriage*, (London, 1938) pp 41-57
(28) *Gentleman's Magazine*, 1810, p. 81.
(29) Hugh Downman, *Infancy or the Management of Children*, (Edinburgh, 1788), p.76.
(30) Ibid p.132
(31) Hugh Downman, *Poems to Thespia*, (Exeter, 1796), p.160.
(32) *Essays by a Society of Gentlemen in Exeter*, (Exeter, 1796). A copy is in the Devon and Exeter Institution.
(33) Richard Polwhele (1760-1838), author of *The History of Devonshire* and The *History of Cornwall* and much else; curate of Kenton 1782-1793; a close friend of Hugh Downman and John Andrew (1750-1799), rector of Powderham and son of John Andrew, the physician; Downman and Andrew were brothers-in-law.
John Sheldon F.R.S. (1752-1808), Professor of Anatomy at the Royal Academy in succession to William Hunter, whose assistant he was. As an anatomist he was considered the best teacher of his generation. He had wide-ranging interests but was mentally somewhat unstable. See *DNB*
For Isaac d'Israeli see *DNB* and Notes and Queries, 5th series, V, p.508.

CHAPTER VIII
Patients' Perspectives

It is pertinent to ask how Thomas Glass was viewed by his patients rather than by his peers; as Roy Porter has pointed out, they have often been given little more than a passing nod in traditional medical biography, or totally ignored.[1] Certain parts of the country are rich in contemporary diaries, often containing piquant medical comment, but such as are held by the Devon Record Office regretably contain nothing relevant to Glass himself; one is forced therefore to clutch at such straws as may by chance present themselves. These are in the form of letters, either to or from Thomas, or between other parties about him.

On December 20, 1744, there is a letter addressed to Thomas Glass by Nick Peters. As he signs himself 'Junior', and refers to his father having been consulted, he was undoubtedly the son of Nicholas Peters, the Topsham apothecary, to whom Samuel had been apprenticed, and who had produced the English translation of the *Commentaries*. He was also an apothecary.[2]

> Sir
>
> *I am exceedingly obliged to you for yesterdays kind message, but as my wife was then better there was no occasion for troubling you and as she still mends I hope there will be no occasion. I suppose my father told you that she had been down stairs above a week & seemed tolerable till last Tuesday seven night. The manner of her first seizure was her awaking in a great hurry, abt 7 in ye morn: soon follow'd a faintness & great oppression of spirits, in order to shake it off shed come down stairs, but it continued all day; she had a good night but it returned again in ye morning, & continued till 6 in ye evening, it then abated, and abt 9 went off without any sweat, nor was ye coming on attended with any shiverings but a numbness in ye Legs with coldness; sometimes she wd have 2 or 3 of these returns in a day & sometimes be free from 'em 24 hrs, without any regularity. When she was first seiz'd I gave her a Vomit, & a few Cordial medicines, at length I came to ye Bark & gave it in substance with a warm draft after. This vomited and purged within half an hour. In ye evening I washed out her Stomach again (this was Friday last), & next morn_ repeated ye Bark, it had ye same Effect, vomited in half an hour & purged. I then stopt it & gave her some Astringents with Cordials, for ye purging tho' not very violent, had prodigiously weakened her. Still these faintings & lowness of spirits continued wth ye usual remissions, till last monday, when she was seiz'd with a paroxysm, much like ye grand one in ye first place, only without ye intermitting pulse, this continued from 3 in ye*

*morning till 6 at night when it went off in a most violent sweat which
lasted near an hour, & after was better than she had been for a week
before. I examined ye neck & breast & found 5 or 6 pretty large miliary
bladders, with a few pimples here & there. Seeing such a fair Interval,
& ye Eruption too, I was doubtful how to proceed, but fearing ye
Consequence of another such paroxysm, I immediately gave ye Extract
of Bark oz 1/2 in pills every 4 hours. Tuesday she was tolerable all day,
yesterday a gentle Return, today better. I'm now in hopes she'll once
more weather ye point, & must desire of you a method how to proceed
after these Intermissions are quite over, for till then ye Bark, perhaps
some time afterward, must be continued in some shape or other. I beg
pardon for giving you this trouble & am Sir*

yr most humble servant

The acute intermittent nature of the fever and the presence of pimples and
miliary bladders, suggests that she was suffering from miliary fever, which
did not always occur in epidemic form.[3]

In February, 1778, a young man of twenty-four, in the company of his sister,
Betsey, went to Exeter to consult Thomas Glass; he was in the late stages of
consumption, impoverished owing to the irresponsible behaviour of his
father, but also notable as the nephew of Sir Joshua Reynolds, being the eldest
of the seven children of Elizabeth Johnson, one of Reynolds's two sisters. The
young man's name was Samuel, born at Torrington in 1754. He left a series
of letters to his mother and sisters, which indicate that his health was beginning to fail in March, 1776. Samuel was staying at Torrington when Betsey
came down from London to be with him; it had been suggested that
Torrington air was bad for him and an opinion was to be sought from Dr
Glass as to the possible advantage of Plymouth.[4]

His symptoms were familiar ones, ebbing strength, strange fits of heat and
cold, night sweats, hacking cough, and an inability to digest his food. He
wrote home from Exeter on 7th February, 1778:

*My dear Mother and Sisters,
I have but a short letter to write you now, the next I hope will be more
satisfactory. It is impossible to tell you yet what effect the journey will
have, as I am sometimes better and sometimes worse, but I am in hopes
that it will take a good turn, and if it does it must do me infinite service.
I have been hitherto better by day and worse by night, but last night
better than the night before. Dr Glass has given me leave to go to
Plymouth, He said it was a damp, foggy place, and damps were not
good for me, but however, said He, try it. I told him I was entirely at his
direction, and if he thought any other place better would comply with
his advice. He said he could not tell where to advise me to go, I ought*

to be near the Seaside tho' not quite close to it, because he said at this time of year those fogs and damps are continually arising from it at all places. Torrington he said would never do for me, the air was too sharp, I must be out of that at all events. He repeated again that he would have me try Plymouth, you can leave it, said He, if you find it does not suit you. So now we are setting out for Oakhampton in the return chaise at half fare, and tomorrow hope to be in Plymouth.

Yr. Dutiful and Affecte Son and Brother
S.Johnson.

Love and Compliments to all friends and enquirers. Dr Glass wrote me a prescription which he hoped would remove my complaint, but I could not press a fee upon him. He said I was very welcome to his advice.

Mr. Daniel Johnson was brother to Samuel's ne'er-do-well father, William, and a surgeon at Torrington; on February 9, Samuel wrote from Plymouth as follows:

Dear Uncle,
I will give you as good an account of myself as I can. On Thursday at Hatherleigh I found myself quite hungry, and ventur'd upon a young chick for dinner. All the evening much better, not the least fatigued, went to bed with good spirits. But alas! no sooner was I laid down than I was seized with a burning heat, which continued all night. I believe I slept about half an hour (I eat nothing but milk for supper). Dr Glass suppos'd this heat proceeded from the animal food or the exercise. It was the latter, for the next day I ate no animal food, but when I went to bed this heat return'd, preceded by violent tremblings; but this did not prevent my sleeping; I slept soundly till my old enemy, one that never leaves me, I mean my Night-Sweats, attack'd me, and prevented me from reaping the benefits of this whole night's sleep.
I got to Exeter about 4; Dr Glass enquir'd of the usual state of my pulse, of which I could give him no information; however He said they were quicker than they ought to be.
Saturday we returned to Oakhampton. I ate whiting for dinner, for Dr Glass said I might venture on those innocent things if I found they agreed with me. That night no heat, and should have slept, I suppose, the whole night, but for the Night-Sweats.
Tuesday we din'd at Tavistock and slept, and this morning arriv'd at Plymouth after five days' journey. After eating a hearty dinner of both fish and fowl, I walk'd out for the first time since I left Torrington, took a boat with the Ladies, it was a fine afternoon, and went aboard the Godfrey, lying about two miles off, to see my Brother Richard. We left him weighing Anchor, and I suppose he is now sail'd.[5]
We are now return'd to give an Account of ourselves to all our friends. For my part I cannot conclude what to make of myself, I am in the most

111

unsettled state in the world, I feel an hundred different symptoms in the day, which I cannot tell what to make of or describe, and am still as weak as a child and as thin as a rush. Walking up and down stairs is sometimes the utmost of my strength. Whether the journey has done me good or harm I do not expect to be able to tell you till I have settled here some days. I have sent you Dr Glass's Prescription, and should be very glad to know what you judge He supposes my disorder to be. You will be kind enough to send me enough for a week by Simon Down, who will see the letter I wrote my Mother, and I wish you would show her this at the same time.

Samuel's last letter was undated, but written at the end of February, 1778; he was unable to finish it , but handed over to his sister:

My dear Mother and Sisters,
As John Yonge has been so very obliging as to offer to come to Plymouth to conduct me home, I write this on purpose to tell him that nothing will give me greater happiness than to see him here the beginning of next week. If he comes on Monday, Simon Down can take back his horse the tuesday morning, and he can return in our chaise.
I am at present in a most doleful (tho' not dangerous) case. I have been for these three days and nights most grievously afflicted with a violent Diarrhoea, which will neither let me rest night nor day, so you may guess how weak I am. All this day and part of yesterday I have been waiting for an Apothecary, but he has been unfortunately not to be met with. I dread this night, but I do not dread the consequences, for all my other complaints are better. My Cough is almost entirely gone, and what is surprizing my Appetite continues so good that I eat my meat quite hungry...

If Samuel did not recognize the true nature of his illness (or subconsciously denied it), Betsey reveals her suspicions in completing the second part of the letter:

it has reduced him to so weak a state that he is not able to walk up or down stairs, and I am exceedingly alarmed at it, as I think I have heard that it is the last complaint that people in consumtions have, you cannot think how miserable it makes me, John Y. can never be a more welcome visitor than he will be both to my brother and me just at this time, as we don't know whether we are acting right or wrong in anything that we do. Mr Madge is not well enough to visit his patients, he has an assistant who always visits them and reports to him their disorders, but that would not be satisfactory to us...[6]

So the matter drew to its ineviteable conclusion, the anecdote illustrates that Thomas Glass did not turn away a manifestly hopeless case, nor would he accept a fee.

112

In another professional encounter in 1770 there is a letter to the patient from Thomas;[7] the full medical history is not available but one may guess from the letter that the symptoms included rheumatic pains, shortness of breath, and cough. The patient was a man of some importance, Alexander, Lord Polwarth, son of Hugh Hume, third Earl of Marchmont; Marchmont was a politician and man about town, close friend and executor of Alexander Pope and known to Boswell and Dr Johnson. Polwarth died in 1781 at the age of 32, eleven years after this letter, which evidently follows a previous consultation:

Exeter, November 1, 1770.

My Lord
Your Lordship will be presently convinced that too favorable a report has been made to You of my Abilities, but such as they are I shall be happy if I can suggest any thing that can contribute to the reestablishment of Your Health; wh. being already so far advanced that scarce any one of Your late complaints remains, & every appearance as favorable as can be wished, was I as a physician to recommend to Your Lordship a change of Situations, whilst You continue to feel Yourself growing better & better every day, I should do it against my Judgement. But if on the nearer approach of winter, Your rheumatic pains should return, or Your breathing become less free & easy, or Your cough should increase, or you feel Yourself not quite so well as You have been, it may then, I think, be adviseable for You to remove to a warmer part of the Kingdom, where You may be exposed as little as possible to dry, thin, cold air. For it is a matter of experience that such a constitution of the air is productive of an inflammatory state of the Blood & its vessels, wh. is naturally follow'd by rheumatic complaints, cough, pains of the side, & Breast, & inflammation of the Lungs; & that those who occupy a low moist country, are less affected by this kind of Distemper than the neighbouring Inhabitants of highlands. The very moist Air of Egypt, bordering on the Nile, & annually overflowed by it, was, when the learned Arts were in the most flourishing State at Rome, recommended by their Physicians to the Italians, who were consumptive, as we learn from Celsus, whose words I beg leave to transcribe, Opus est, si vires patiuntur, caeli mutatione, sic ut densius quam id est, ex quo discedit aeger, petatur: ideoque aptissime Alexandriam ex Italia itur.
[If strength allows, a change of air is necessary, such that a denser climate should be sought than that from which the patient has come; hence the most suitable is the voyage to Alexandria from Italy][8]

For the above reason, if Your Lordship should think proper to remove from your own Houses, I wish one may be found in this part of the country, fit to receive Yourself & family, situated in a fertile valley, at

113

a due distance from the Sea, not too near any high Hills, & beyond the reach of any noxious Effluvia from marshy ground. What makes it difficult to procure a convenient House in such a situation in these parts, is that this country is generally hilly, & that there are few gentlemens seats, but what are inhabited by their owners or families during the winter. In the mean time I shall desire some friends to enquire if such a one is to be procured, & am wh. the greatest respect,
Your Lordships
Most obedient humble Servant

The connection between Lord Polwarth and the West of England is not immediately apparent, though his father, Lord Marchmont almost certainly knew Ralph Allen, through their mutual friendship with Alexander Pope. Ralph Allen was president of the Devon and Exeter Hospital in 1758, and a substantial benefactor.[9] Polwarth's grandfather, then Sir Patrick Hume, had been a supporter of William of Orange, was present at Torbay when he landed in 1688, and accompanied him on his march to London. From the contents of the letter to Lord Polwarth there seems little doubt that he too was a sufferer from consumption, that which John Bunyan called 'The captain of all the men of death'.

The last letter was written to Mrs. Melina (Melony) Daniell, Thomas Glass's youngest daughter, by Francis Coleman, on January 5, 1802.[10] It was in connection with a portrait of her father, which he had just sent to her. The portrait was painted by Hudson in about 1750 and had been commissioned by Henry Cruwys of Hillersdon as a mark of gratitude for medical attention received from Thomas.[11] Francis Coleman had been a friend of Henry Cruwys and had acquired Hillersdon from him:

Dear Madam,
When I last had the pleasure of seeing that excellent man your father, at Hillersdon, upon my telling him that I had at that time some thought of disposing of that house, it drew from him, I well remember, this observation - should a king arise in Egypt who knew not Joseph, would I have the goodness, looking steadfastly at his own picture, to give it either to him or to one of his family. This I have ever since treasured up in my mind, and the time is now arrived by my parting with Hillersdon when I can with pleasure fulfil my intention by requesting your acceptance of it. I can assure I ever looked with pleasure on the portrait of a man that was not only an honour to his country, and his profession but as it was also a testimony of gratitude from my old friend Mr. Cruwys to your father, to whose skill and attention, he more than once considered himself indebted for his life. I must now beg to thank you for your very handsome letter upon this occasion and with my wife's united best

114

compliments believe me
Madam, your very obedient humble servant

There were at that time only two surviving daughters, of which Melony was the youngest; she dutifully passed the portrait on to Ann, married to John Lowder and living in Bath.

Notes

(1)   Roy Porter, *Patients and Practioners*, (Cambridge, 1985), p.2.
(2)   D.R.O. 72/1/2/1
(3)   For miliary fever see note 22, Chapter IV.
(4)   Susan M. Radcliffe (ed.), *Sir Joshua's Nephew*, (London, 1930), pp. 228-236. It would seem that Reynolds does not emerge with great credit from this story, apparently treating his sister with little generosity, destitute as she was, with seven children.
(5)   Samuel's brother, Richard, went out to India, embarking at Plymouth just before Samuel's death.
(6)   Mr. Madge is probably Dr John Mudge (1721-1793), of Plymouth, see Chapter II, note 10.
(7)   British Library, Add 35384 ff 352-352 by permission of the British Library.
(8)   The passage is from Celsus, *De Medicina*, Book III. 22. 8, which deals with chronic phthisis.
(9)   For references to Hugh Hume, Lord Marchmont, see DNB Maynard Mack, *Alexander Pope. A Life* (New Haven, 1985), passim, and James Boswell, The Life of Samuel Johnson, (London, 1901), passim. Alexander was the son of Lord Hume's second wife, Elizabeth Crompton, whom he married in 1748. He was a lifelong friend of Alexander Pope, a possible link in the chain between Thomas Glass, Ralph Allen, and his son. Ralph Allen is referred to by Maynard Mack, op. cit.
Unfortunately Pope quarrelled with Allen in 1743. Allen also was known well to Fielding who cast him as Squire Allworthy in *Tom Jones*. His link with the Devon and Exeter Hospital is referred to by J. Delpratt Harris, *The Royal Devon and Exeter Hospital*, (Exeter, 1922), pp.37-39. His portrait by William Hoare is still at the hospital.
Henry Fielding had probably been known to Thomas Glass in his youth, since he had enrolled as a student in the faculty of Letters at the University of Leyden in 1728, the year that Thomas began his studies, remaining until August 1729.
(10) The letter and the portrait were handed down to Lancelot Lowder, Ann's great grandson, who was killed at the battle of Loos in 1915. They then passed to the descendants of Mary Parminter, and are now in the possession of Lord Borthwick, of Crookston, Midlothian.
(11) Henry Cruwys, a member of a very ancient Devon family, with their seat at Cruwys Morchard, near Tiverton. W.G. Hoskins, however, says that the hackneyed jingle in which this name appears has not a word of truth in it. See *Devon*, (London, 1964; Exeter 1992), p. 76.

CHAPTER IX

Influenza and Other Epidemics in Exeter

The unpublished edition of Celsus.
The Leyden Dissertation

As far as London was concerned, the medical scene was dominated by the Royal College of Physicians for the first seventy-one years of the eighteenth century. The college operated a form of medical freemasonry, whereby the narrow path to the top of this exclusive fraternity was denied to all but members of the established church, and made very difficult for any who had graduated anywhere but Oxford or Cambridge. As far as provincial physicians were concerned this did not present a problem, but there were a number of very able physicians in London, such as John Fothergill and William Hunter, who felt themselves frozen out by the system. In about 1752 a group of these formed themselves into a Medical Society, whose members were invited to read papers before it; these were published, at Fothergill's expense, as *Medical Observations and Enquiries*; they were essays of considerable clinical importance, six volumes being issued between 1757 and 1784.[1] One of the many topics Fothergill selected for scrutiny was the countrywide influenza epidemic of 1775; he himself described the illness as it presented in London and he asked Thomas Glass to describe the epidemic as he saw it in Exeter. In fact the essay did not appear until 1784, in the sixth volume of the series.[2]

Speaking at first of Epidemical Colds, Thomas did not use the word influenza until towards the end of the piece, saying that it was a word coined in Italy, literally 'influence of the stars', a relic of the times when it was the general opinion of philosophers that all things on earth were governed by the heavens; it was probably what had been called Tussis Epidemica by Sydenham, and Febris Catarrhalis Epidemica by his predecessors.

As far as Exeter was concerned, the illness struck about November 8, about a week after it appeared in London, and had all but vanished by December 4:

> *On the 11th or 12th of November it made its appearance in the Devon and Exeter Hospital, and within a week seized 173 persons, being all the servants and patients then in the house, except two children; 162 of them coughing together. Is it not remarkable that such a number of hospital patients, afflicted with so various and different kinds of distem-*

pers, and under the operations of the most efficacious medicines of the most opposite qualities, should have been all affected, almost at the same time, and in the same manner, by the cause of these epidemical coughs?

Two or three days after the hospital had been attacked, the City Workhouse was visited by them [it]: of near 200 poor people, who are in this house, but few escaped; all the others were complaining at the same time.

The condition had spread throughout Devon and Cornwall by the end of the first week of December, seldom lasting more than three to four weeks:

Its appearance in this city was the same as in London, except only, that it was here much more favourable, and attended with some symptoms besides those you have mentioned in your Sketch: for many of our patients, especially such as had a considerable degree of fever, complained of great lowness of spirits and sudden weakness; several of them of a perfect inappetency both to meat and drink (most of these had severe coughs without much fever), and some a soreness throughout the windpipe and oesophagus, with a great pain in swallowing even liquids, others of a violent pain in their ears. A few had sloughs of a malignant kind on their tonsils; swelling of these, and of the submaxillary glands were not unfrequent, but occurred oftener in some towns than in others. One of my patients had a large parotid, which suppu-

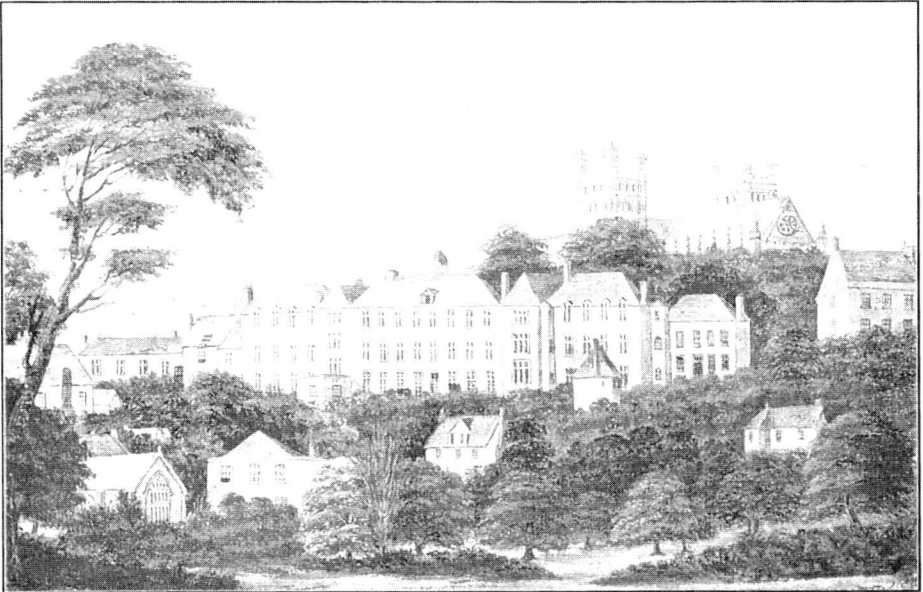

Devon and Exeter Hospital, 1852, by John Harris.

117

rated slowly, and broke at the end of three weeks. Eruptions on the lips,
towards the crisis, were a common and very salutary symptom. Many
felt no feverish heat, but almost all, if not all, had more or less of a
cough.

The great majority needed no particular treatment, but those who were
feverish or had pains in head, back, breast or limbs, were advised by the
Faculty in Exeter to confine themselves to their beds, and to drink frequently
barley water, water gruel, linseed tea, and other soft diluting liquors, which
were sometimes sweetened with honey, very hot:

> *A plentiful and easy sweat, continued for a sufficient space of time,*
> *carried off the catarrhous fever and pains on the first, second, third, or*
> *fourth day of the disease. This fever, which has been called a Diary and*
> *Decreasing Fever, because it either ends or begins to decline within*
> *twenty-four hours,and never exceeds the fourth day, was accounted an*
> *essential part of the Catarrhous Epidemic, and seems indeed to be an*
> *immediate effect of its cause.*
>
> *... In a certain town, many persons to whom, as soon as they applied for*
> *assistance, wine whey with spirits of hartshorn was freely given to force*
> *out a sweat, and paregoric elixir to quiet their cough, became delirious.*
> *Sometimes a violent cough, with considerable but not inflammatory*
> *pains about the breast, seemed to require bleeding on the second or third*
> *day of the disease; but this evacuation weakened the patient, without*
> *mitigating his cough in any considerable degree, and seemed to retard*
> *his recovery.*

Since the loss of blood seemed in some cases to bring on severe bouts of intermittent fever, he concluded that bleeding in this distemper should be
employed only when it was accompanied by real inflammatory symptoms; in
most cases all that was required was a proper regimen. This was after all the
experience of 'our sagacious Sydenham' who cured the Stationary Fever of
1675, when it was united with the Epidemical Cough of that year, in the same
manner and with the same success, as he had done before these coughs made
their appearance.

Thus far, the management of influenza seems almost that of the twentieth
century in its restraint from intervention; the introduction of the concept of
the 'atrabilious constitution', a Boerhaavian favourite, may have been more
controversial:[3]

> *Before we were visited by the late Epidemic, the atrabilious constitu-*
> *tion, which according to Dr Grant's accurate observations, begins some*
> *time in October, or the beginning of November, had taken place. And*
> *on this account a plentiful discharge of black bilious stools, coming on*
> *of its own accord, or procured by gentle and repeated purging medi-*
> *cines, when there were pains or uneasiness in the bowels, or a disten-*

sion of the belly and praecordia, with inquietude or other signs of turgid matter in the intestines, soon freed the patient from the fever of the season, and all the complaints arising from it.

If there were inflammatory complaints, and blood was taken away, it was always sizy;[4] likewise recourse was sometimes taken to antiphlogistic medicines, and occasionally to blisters, which were more effective in relieving pleuritic pains than bleeding:

Peripneumonic complaints, the most alarming symptom of all, were gradually carried off by a free and easy expectoration of digested matter. Such remedies were therefore administered, as have been found by experience, to promote the digestion of thick viscid humours, collected and retained in the lungs, and to facilitate their discharge.

This all seems to indicate a modification of the writer's previous somewhat heroic approach to fevers. In all it had been fatal to only a very few in this part of the country, and those who died of it were 'ancient persons or pulmonics'.

In discussing causation, Thomas stressed that the epidemic could not be related to moist, cold weather, as Wintringham and others had stated, since there were many historical records of severe outbreaks at all seasons. He adds his own observation, that, contrary to general opinion, the distemper did not seem to arise from contagion:

For in this city, in the year 1729, it was conjectured that two thousand persons at least were seized with it in one night. But what is more extraordinary, before the beginning of autumn, in the year 1557, it attacked all parts of Spain at once, so that the greatest part of the people in that kingdom were seized with it almost on the same day.

In all, said Thomas, we were no nearer establishing a cause than were the ancient Greeks, who ascribed it to something in the air, undetectable by the senses, or reasonably, by Hippocrates, to God. For what it was worth, he added that in this area many horses and dogs were severely afflicted with colds and cough in the month of September, something that had been observed in three general epidemics that had happened within recent times.

John Huxham, at Plymouth, had been keeping regular weather records since 1724, at the instigation of James Jurin, one of the secretaries of the Royal Society. In addition, in parallel with these, he kept monthly records of the prevalence of epidemic diseases between 1728 and 1748. In 1733 he gave a wonderfully perceptive description of an influenza epidemic, though he did not name it, which started on February 10. Ten years later he reported another outbreak, saying that the fever seemed to have been identical with that rife in Europe, and termed the influenza.[5]

The Exeter physicians, from time to time, considered it necessary to allay public anxiety by issuing statements to the press about current epidemics:

Exeter Flying Post, *29th May, 1767.*
It being generally reported and believed that there has for some time raged and continues to rage in this City, an infectious Fever: we think it our duty to assure the Public that such Report is false and groundless. It is true that about six weeks since some Persons were seized with a dangerous Fever of whom however we cannot find that more than twelve have died; and it is our firm Opinion and Belief that the City has seldom been more healthy than it is at present.

John Andrew MD   Tho. Glass MD
Geo. Bent MD   S. Musgrave M.D

Or this:

Exeter Flying Post, *30th October, 1779.*
To satisfy the Public that the alarming account inserted in the London Evening Post, on the 16th instant, as well as in several other newspapers of a SCARLET FEVER raging at Exeter, with a fatality peculiar to PLAGUE, is an absolute Falsehood, invented and conveyed to every part of the Kingdom by one of those Wretches who delight in doing mischief to injure this City and to add to our Natural Calamities the frightful apprehension of the Plague being broke out among us. We presume the simple Relation of the following Matters of Fact will be fully sufficient.

By a Survey of the City and Suburbs of Exeter, executed but not with the utmost exactness in the year 1774, the Inhabitants were found to be near 20,000. The Number of Burials at a Medium for the twenty preceding years was 500.

In the year 1777 it was found by careful Enquiry made of every family that 1850 persons were taken with the Small Pox in the natural way; that of these 275 died, which is very near one in Seven.

From the Beginning of the present year 1779 to the 20th inst. 1666 persons have had the contagious Fever, which is usually attended with a Scarlet Appearance on the Skin, and a soreness of the throat, of which 72 have died, which is about one in twenty -three.

This Numeration is made from the Accounts we have been favoured with by our Apothecaries; every one of them having given us the Number of their Patients, which on examining his Books he found he had visited, and of those he had lost in our reigning Epidemic.

Let it be observed that every poor Person of this City who wants the Assistance of an Apothecary has it readily given him on his applying for it.

The Number of Burials this present Year, to the 25th October, has been 448.

The Proportional Number for that Time, taken from the Accounts of former years, (as above mentioned) is nearly 417, so that the excess of the Number of Burials for this Period is only 31.

Tho. Glass Rob. Harvey	}
Tho. Okes Barth. Parr	}Physicians in Exeter
Tho. Ruston	}

That this could happen, would seem to indicate that the physicians could act together as a group for the civic good, and also that even the poorest could call on the services of an apothecary.

Another letter appeared in the *Flying Post* from a physician at Plymouth, styling himself *Humanus*, in which he refers to the 'very learned and ingenious Dr Glass, who is so deservedly celebrated throughout Europe':

Exeter Flying Post, *8th August, 1777.*

'would save a Life
Rather than wear a Crown'
Downman's *Infancy*

The Measles are now raging in several parts of this County and many fall Victims to their Fury. It is the Duty of every Man to contribute as much as lies in his power to the Preservation of his Species; and He who thinks he is acquainted with any Method to obtain that desirable End, and does not make it as generally known as he is able, is a bad Member of Society. ... To avoid this Imputation, I shall be obliged to you, if you would give a Place in your Paper to the following Method of Treatment of the Measles, with which many of the Faculty, I apprehend, are unacquainted.

A common and dangerous Attendant upon this Disorder is a Peripneumony, and notwithstanding the most judicious Application of the Means generally apply'd, the Lungs are frequently inflamed, and Death is the consequence. ... The Method I would advise is that during the Eruption the Patient should have 3 or 4 Stools given him every Day, which may be procured by directing a Saline Draught cü Sp. Ceti, to be taken every six hours, with as much Pulv. Laxant. added to each as will answer that End. ... I have known Children who have not been known to be prevail'd upon to take Draughts of the above Kind, daily drink Sena [sic] tea suffiucient for the purpose. ... Numbers have I seen treated in this Method and all with the greatest success. ... The Eruption (which is no critical Discharge but merely Symptomatical) has not in the least been check'd, and the Fever and Cough have both

been lessen'd; I never saw any peripneumonic Affection, and conse-
quently no Necessity for Bleeding, and the Cough has soon altogether
disappear'd. ... It is well known that sometimes Nature herself abates
the Fever, and other symptoms of the Measles, by a mild Diarrhoea. ...
I have seen a Mixt. cü Mucilag: Gum Tragacanth sometimes directed,
which could be serviceable only by allaying any irritation in the Throat,
and Pectoral Decoct. order'd to be drank, ... but everyone conversant in
Practice knows that very little is to be expected from Diluting Liquors
when children (the most common subjects of this Disease) are the
Patients; as the quantity they drink is very inconsiderable.

A Friend of Exeter communicated to me the above Method (which
certainly is a great acquisition) about three years ago, and then told me
we are indebted for it to the very learned and ingenious Dr Glass, who
is so deservedly celebrated throughout Europe.

I am, Sir, your most humble Servant
Humanus

It was to be many many years before that old medical trap, embodied in '*post hoc ergo propter hoc*' was to be fully accepted.

Thomas Glass's unpublished edition of Celsus

In 1762, Thomas commenced his major written work, which mysteriously was never published; as far as Exeter was concerned, the work had disappeared from 1848 until 1991, when it became apparent that it had been sleeping in the interval in the Bodleian Library, in four bulky volumes.[6]

The existence of this manuscript was revealed by Bartholemew Parr in his *Anecdotes*:

> *the three volumes of his Celsus with notes have never been printed. I*
> *read them some years since, but dare not from recollection offer any*
> *opinion of their merit. They will be found probably more useful in a*
> *philological, than a medical view, for to connect the Doctrines of Celsus*
> *with those of modern Practitioners, requires a greater extent of knowl-*
> *edge than Dr Glass possessed.*

Again, displaying a wayward ambivalence after several less than generous paragraphs, he concludes:

> *As affording materials for a new edition of Celsus, if my memory*
> *properly assists me, and in this I have the concurrence of a judicious*
> *Friend, to whom the volumes were once communicated, Dr Glass's*
> *Labours would have been highly useful; and I may express my wishes*
> *that they may yet be employed for this purpose.*

Dr George Daniell (1760-1822) was elected physician to the hospital in 1786. In January, 1813, he wrote to the committee urging the formation of a library for the staff, and for those medical gentlemen who practised in the city who do not form a portion of the hospital staff.[7] Presumably with the approval of the cathedral authorities, all or almost all of Thomas Glass's large collection of books, bequeathed to the cathedral, was removed to the Devon and Exeter Hospital in 1814, not to be returned until 1948. The manuscripts were not to be found in the Glass collection of medical books, so carefully catalogued and cherished in Exeter Cathedral library; a chance encounter with a dusty catalogue of 1877, of the Radcliffe Science library, provided the clue that the manuscripts had found their way to Oxford.

Speculation as to how this happened is not necessary; for on the flyleaf of the first and last volumes it may be seen that they were presented by John Bampfylde Daniell MD, an Oxford graduate, in 1848. He was George Daniell's son; the manuscripts had, it seems, either been given to him by his father or left to him when he died in 1822. He practised in London, so had few direct links with Exeter.

One may however ask oneself how Dr George Daniell acquired the manuscripts. The least charitable explanation is that he extracted them from the library for 'safekeeping'; the more likely is that they were given to him by Thomas, who hoped that in some way they would achieve posthumous publication. Thomas was related to George by marriage; his youngest daughter, Melony, had married Samuel Daniell, his brother. George, the young physician, joined the hospital in 1786, the year that Thomas was elected President of the hospital, when his health was fast failing.

The manuscripts are in four volumes and relate to the first four books of *De re Medica (De Medicina)* by Celsus, specifically the Rotterdam edition of 1750 (*cura et studio* Th. J. ab Almeloveen). The first three volumes systematically examine and expand on sections of the text, which constantly refers back to the classical authors; not only medical and scientific, but literary ones as well. It refers also to comment and annotations by other writers such as Caesarius, Constantine, and Scaliger, printed in the previous edition (Leyden, 1746), so that all statements made by Celsus are subjected to very careful scrutiny; the whole is written in Latin, except where there is reference to Greek texts and here the script is Greek. Thirteen pages of introductory notes are followed by 640 pages of commentary, with meticulous references, including those to ten previous editions of Celsus from 1478 (Florentine) to 1746 (Leyden).

The fourth volume contains the detached pages of the actual printed book, remounted between pages of the manuscript book, on which detailed marginal notes and coded references have been made, largely of a philological or grammatical nature; there is also an index.

In Exeter Cathedral library there is a copy of the Leyden edition of Celsus of 1746, in two volumes; each volume is marked on the flyleaf: 'Prepared for a new edition of Celsus by Dr Glass.' There are very similar marginal annotations to those in the fourth volume of the Bodleian manuscripts, but whereas those are immaculate, the Exeter ones are not; there are frequent deletions, emendations, ink blots and water stains. Thomas was evidently not satisfied with this earlier exercise and abandoned it.

There are a number of different editions of Celsus in the medical section of Exeter cathedral library, the oldest being the Venetian incunabulum edition of 1497. A mystery attaches to another which belonged to Thomas, the Parisian edition of 1529, mentioned specifically in the Bodleian manuscripts. This bears the signature J. Letherland, 1745, and Thomas implied that it had previously been owned by Richard Mead; Letherland was physician to Queen Charlotte. This book was present in 1947, being mentioned specifically by the then librarian, Marjorie Crichton, but is not now in the collection, nor was it when the collection was recatalogued in the recent past.[8]

It is significant that only the first four volumes of the total eight in the work were selected; those dealing with clinical medicine and excluding those on pharmacology and surgery. Was there any particular motive in this very substantial piece of writing, other than the furtherance of knowledge? In 1776 Thomas, along with other notables was elected a Foreign Associate of the Royal Society of Medicine of Paris. Parr stated in 1795:

> *Yet this compliment was received with peculiar complacency, was followed by no literary Exertions; and no contribution to the Society followed.*
> *The Commentary on Celsus which had been for some time finished, was designed for this new Society, and to be printed at their Expence. I know not whether it was offered; but it certainly made no part of their Plan, and the offer, if made, must have been declined.*

However it clearly states on the Bodleian manuscript, on the last page of the introduction, that the commentary was written (or at least commenced) in 1762, fourteen years before the French chose to honour him, so why the long interval? And why was the book never published?

Thomas Glass's Inaugural Dissertation at Leyden

Atrophy in general, Phthisis of the Lungs, and those Particular Diseases which lead to it. [*Atrophia in genere, phthisi pulmonali, morbisque praecipuis, qui in eam tendunt.*].

No doubt Thomas would very many times in his life be reminded of his youthful description of the sufferer *in extremis:*

> *foetid breath, pain in the chest, sore nipples, exacerbated by coughing, and more difficulty in breathing every day; hectic fever, noticeably*

124

DISSERTATIO MEDICA

INAUGURALIS

DE

ATROPHIA IN GENERE, PHTHISI PULMONALI, MORBIS- QUE PRÆCIPUIS, QUI IN EAM TENDUNT.

QVAM

ANNUENTE DEO TER OPT. MAX.

Ex Auctoritate Magnifici Rectoris,

D. PETRI BURMANNI,

J.U.D. HISTORIARUM, GRÆCÆ LINGUÆ, ELOQUENTIÆ,
POETICES, ET HISTORIÆ FOEDERATI BELGII,
PROFESSORIS, UT ET BIBLIOTHECARII,

NEC NON

Amplissimi SENATUS ACADEMICI *Consensu,*

ET

Nobilissimae FACULTATIS MEDICAE *Decreto,*

PRO GRADU DOCTORATUS,

Summisque in MEDICINA Honoribus &
Privilegiis ritè ac legitimè consequendis,
Eruditorum Examini submittit

THOMAS GLASS, Anglo-Britannus.

Ad diem 13. Julii 1731.
hora locoque solitis.

LUGDUNI BATAVORUM,
Apud JOANNEM LUZAC, 1731.

Title page of Tomas Glass's Leyden dissertation.

worse at night and fading by first light, with a weak slow pulse and warmth in the upper parts from the acridity, lips and face becoming flushed; there is great thirst and sweating at night, extreme anxiety coincides with the time the fever starts and a host of misfortunes follow; there is total wasting away of the body, flesh vanishes and bony articulations and processes protrude everywhere; the nails are incurved and the facies described by Hippocrates is plain to see (thus did Aretaeus so vividly depict the image of death); the feet swell, and sometimes the hands, there is great weakness and red pustules and hoarse voice may be present.

It is perhaps too easy to assume that Thomas's inaugural dissertation was entirely his own work, it is more than possible that the guiding hand of his professor at least pointed the way; but, whatever the truth, it provides a digest of received teaching in the realm of physiology, in what was to become known as pathology, in clinical medicine, and in therapeutics.

In that sense there was nothing innovative about the essay, but it extended to some thirteen thousand words and, if it does seem somewhat repetitive at times to our ears, it is a work of some substance, demonstrating keenness of observation and an imaginative turn of phrase:

whence yellow Diarrhoea, foetid, purulent, becoming liquid as sputum diminishes; almost always this opens the doorway to the house of death.

He doffs his cap at frequent intervals to his teachers, to the classical authors, and to more contemporary authorities, such as Malpighi, Leeuenhoek, Hook, and Ruysch, a policy that will be recognised by all writers of doctoral theses, of whatever generation; he also hangs as many hats as possible, metaphorically speaking, on any particular peg.

If there is one name that appears above all others, excluding Boerhaave, it is that of Christopher Bennet (1617-1655), author of *Theatrum Tabidorum*, who himself died early from consumption, that to which all paths seem to lead in this narrative.[9] It may be said too, that many years later, Baron van Swieten in his Commentaries on Boerhaave's Aphorisms, covered the same ground and in the same terms as had Thomas in his youth.[10] Bartholemew Parr was not unkind to Thomas in respect of this early writing, even giving it grudging approval, but implied nevertheless that it was not entirely Thomas's own work:

At Leyden, I apprehend they are, in part, composed by the candidate, modelled and carefully corrected by the Professor; while at Edinburgh they are almost exclusively the work of the Graduate. In this Essay, I perceive that Dr Glass scarcely steps beyond the confines of Boerhaave and Hippocrates, except when he rests on the authority of Bennet, whom Boerhaave also trusted. We seem almost to read the commentaries of Haller and van Swieten, on the Institutions and Aphorisms of

Boerhaave, and to follow the cool, well arranged train of scientifc inves-
tigation from the Pen of a Veteran in Medicine.

Van Swieten himself placed great confidence in the words of Bennet, referring to him very frequently, acknowledging his words to have greater weight because of his own experience as a sufferer. He quoted from the prelude to Bennet's book:

Thou treatest of the phthisis,
Not only from the accounts of authors,
But from thy own sufferings;
And thou wast at the same time
The patient and the physician.
It is not easy to say,
Whether thy disease was more grievous, or
Thy recovery more glorious.

While still in the foothills of his expedition, Thomas dwelt first on the development of the egg, that of the fowl, wherein the carina, the keel, ultimately to become the spine, is laid down as it might be in a shipyard; all the while it is bathed in a nourishing fluid, the albumen, the process in man being identical. Boerhaave himself uses the term carina in this context, speaking at the same time of 'the incipient chick'.[11]

Improper nutrition causes atrophy or wasting conditions, arising first from defects in the chyle, leading to Cacochymia, an unhealthy state of the humours. This sets in train a whole catalogue of ills, of which particular emphasis is given to Acrid catarrh, Cold Pituitous Congestion, Haemoptysis, and finally Phthisis itself.

Intervention by man in this process is wide-ranging, dealing with climate, exercise, diet, hot bathing, bleeding, ligatures, and very extensive application of the *Materia Medica*.

Perhaps it was the impetuousness of youth or the driving force that directed his later working life that led Thomas to choose a topic as challenging as that of consumption; so defeating and yet so enigmatic, a headlong gallop towards disaster or unexpected recovery against all the portents. Of course it was all around: 'Youth grows pale, and spectre thin, and dies'. As Baron van Swieten wrote,[12] anticipating Keats:

How frequently have physicians lamented to see this cruel disease
snatch away, in the flower of their age, beautiful young persons of both
sexes, as a storm beats down roses in their bloom!

Thomas named Gerhard van Swieten amongst his friends at Leyden, though the latter was nine years older. He had continued there as a lecturer, after completing his own studies.

Examination of the candidate at Leyden, when he was required to defend his thesis, was conducted in Latin by the *Rector Magnificus*, in Thomas's case Peter Burmann, in the presence of the *Praeses*, and other professors. It took place on July 13, 1731. His diploma was signed by Burmann, Boerhaave, Oostendijk Schacht (his promoter), and Albinus.[13]

Notes

(1)   The split in the profession, consequent on the elitism of the Royal College, led to a considerable upheaval within its ranks.   This is dealt with very fully by Ivan Waddington,' The Struggle to Reform the Royal College of Physicians, 1767-1771: A Sociological Analysis', *Medical History* 17 (1973), pp. 107-126. R. Hingston Fox, *Dr John Fothergill and his friends*, (London, 1919), pp 143-151, also provides considerable information on this, and on the Medical Society, p.141. Thomas Glass's paper on Influenza is mentioned on pp.71-72

(2)   *Medical Observations and Inquiries*, Vol. VI, (1784), pp.364-377.

(3)   The concept of atrabilis or black bile dates from Hippocrates and was revived by Boerhaave. It had a synonymous association with melancholia. Baron van Swieten, *Commentaries upon Boerhaave's Aphorisms*, (Edinburgh, 1776), Vol. XI, devotes the first 112 pages to this topic. Grant evidently considered that October or early November was the danger time for melancholics.

(4)   The siziness is the thickness of the yellow crust which separates when blood removed from the body has been standing a while.

(5)   For a review of Huxham's life and his two volumes on airs and epidemic diseases, see R.M.S. McConaghey, 'John Huxham', *Medical History* Vol. XIII, No 3, (July, 1969), pp.280-287.

(6)   Bodleian Library reference MS Radcliffe Trust e. 58.

(7)   J. Delpratt Harris, *The Royal Devon and Exeter Hospital*, (Exeter,1922) p. 88.

(8)   Marjorie Crichton, *Transactions of the Devonshire Association*, 1947, p.118. Celsus, though probably not himself a physician, amassed a comprehensive digest of medical and scientific knowledge of the time, probably in the first century AD.

(9)   Bennet was another West Country physician, who practised first in Bristol and then in London. *Theatri Tabidorum vestibulum seu Exercitationes...* was first published in London in 1654, the year before he died. See DNB.

(10) Baron G. van Swieten, *Commentaries upon Boerhaave's Aphorisms*, Vol. XII, (Edinburgh, 1776), p. 108.

(11) Boerhaave, *Institutes of Medicine*, (1742-1746), Vol. 3, pp. 346355.

(12) van Swieten, op. cit., p. 14.

(13) The diploma is in the possession of Lord Borthwick, of Crookston, Midlothian.

CHAPTER X
The Ancient Baths

The Use made of a very hot Bath, was to draw the Humours, as it is done by a CuppingGlass, from the inner Parts of the Body to the outer; to scatter and diffuse the same, when accumulated, extravasated, or stagnating any where, within or below the common integuments;

In 1752 Thomas Glass published, in London, a forty two page tract. This was *An Account of the Antient Baths, and their use in physic.* Thomas revealed a considerable interest in treatment by hot bathing in his inaugural dissertation at Leyden, and continued to be an enthusiast in his more mature years. He first applied himself in his essay, to an historical review of the subject in the classical literature of Greece and Rome. He pointed out, as he had done in his *Twelve Commentaries*, that there were definite disadvantages in the modern view, that macerating in hot water and sweating in bed afterwards would answer all the ends and purposes of bathing; it was a mistake, attended with very bad consequences.

Predictably, with Galen as a starting point, he described how a person would progress through rooms of different temperatures, from *Tepidarium* to *Caldarium*, and thence to *Frigidarium*; the rooms were heated by a kiln or oven underneath, and each room had its own water bath. The bather usually sat down on a low seat in the bath, with legs and sometimes thighs covered, while water was poured on their heads and upper parts.

Thomas allowed himself a certain amount of architectural digression; for example, the younger Pliny's description of certain other types of Roman baths for private, as opposed to public, use, and the precise nature of the hanging baths, or *Balnea pensilia.*

Methods of treating a wide variety of disorders had been described by such as Celsus, Galen, Avicenna, and Asclepiades and the text is rich in graceful Latin.

The effect of the hot air was that all the pores of the body were dilated and opened, especially those parts that were contiguous to it; at the same time the heart and arteries were stimulated to contract more frequently and vigorously:

By means of which the Motion of the Blood will be accelerated, and the Flux of the Humours be more determined towards the Skin and Passages conveying the Breath: For the Arteries nearest these Parts are most stimulated to propel their Fluids, and the Ducts and Pores most open to transmit them: Consequently the Discharge of the useless excrementitious Matter, which naturally passeth off through the perspiratory Pores, will be thereby greatly increased.

... Another Effect of hot Air is fusing and dissolving the Blood and Humours, together with such Concretions as are not too far removed from a fluid State, and disposed to dissolve by Heat; such are Fat, cold Pituita, and crude, viscid Matter. The two last are, for the most Part, the obstructing Matter in those chronical Distempers where the circulation is languid. A general Redundancy of the former is itself a Distemper, and the Cause of many others.

... The general Intent of anointing with sweet Oil in the hot Rooms, was to relax the solid Parts, that the Ducts and Pores might more easily give way to the Humours, which were to pass through them. By rubbing, which was usually done with Oil, the Vessels and Pores were alternately and successively compressed and dilated; the Humours forcibly driven forward and backward, and in all Directions; the component Particles of both Solids and Fluids agitated and impelled against one another: The Consequence must be Increase of Heat, a larger Flux of Humours to the Superficies; Expression of the perspirable Matter in or near the skin ...

... When the Motion of the Blood had been gradually quickened, the gross Humours attenuated, the thick Juices dissolved, the perspiratory Matter discharged, the Vessels unloaded, and the narrower passages opened by the first Part of the Baths; a Person was properly prepared for a greater Rarefaction and Agitation of the Fluids and Solids in the second, which was much hotter than the first.

Switching quite suddenly to the contemporary scene, Thomas warns against rash and sudden exposure to the intense heat of a hot bath, often with fatal results:

by bringing on Fevers, Pleurisies, Inflammations of the Viscera and Apoplexies. To prevent such Accidents, Physicians have now recourse to bleeding, purging, cooling Diet, and attenuating Medicines.[1]

...This Preparation is evidently more tedious and disagreeable than that recommended by our Predecessors, if not less safe.

The physicians at the Devon and Exeter hospital were evidently concerned that no hot and cold water baths and sweating room had been provided, and, following their recommendation, the installation was duly sanctioned by the Governors on October 29, 1751, at a cost of £450.[2] They would scarcely therefore have started functioning at the time that Thomas published his essay in 1752. Because of the lack of facilities at Exeter until this time, patients with palsies or paralytic disorders, who did not respond to conventional management, were sent to Bath for treatment. The regime was described in 1751 by Dr John Summers, of the Bath Infirmary, in *A short account of the success of warm bathing in paralytic disorders.*[3]

As far as the Exeter physicians were concerned one very important form of palsy was that which followed Devon's own serious endemic disorder of those times, the Devonshire colic.

This had been described by Musgrave in 1703,[4] and more fully by Huxham.[5] The latter had noted its tendency to occur in the latter months of the year, connecting it with the cider harvest. He gave a graphic description of the symptoms and there was no doubt that it was a most alarming and often fatal disease. Starting with excruciating abdominal pains, intractable vomiting gave way to to agonies in muscles and bones, and the weakness and subsequent paralysis that brought a fatal conclusion. If recovery occurred the charactistic residual symptom was wrist drop, causing victims to be known, rather unkindly, as 'Danglers'.

The story is well known now, of course, how Dr (later Sir) George Baker in 1767, in one of the most astonishing pieces of inductive medical reasoning, identified the cause as not the cider, but the lead vessels in which the cider was made.[6]

Baker, in his paper, stated that it was John Andrew who provided him with the figures of admissions to the Devon and Exeter Hospital with the colic, from September, 1762 to July, 1767. These totalled 285, of which 209 were cured. Andrew told Baker that the Devon and Exeter patients came from all over the county, but chiefly from those parts where cider was made. The late R.M.S. McConaghey, in his comprehensive paper on this topic,[7] pointed out that the Exeter records for the years covered by Andrew's figures are missing, implying that he omitted to return the records to the hospital office!

Thomas Glass was evidently, in 1752, very interested in comparing the treatment of palsies and paralytic disorders by conventional means at the Devon and Exeter Hospital with those of John Summers, treated at Bath by warm bathing:

> But let me in the mean Time observe, that the Success of warm bathing in paralytic Disorders is not so fully proved, by the Account of Patients admitted into the Bath Infirmary under such Circumstances, as Dr Summers seems to imagine. And this, I presume, will appear, on comparing that Account with the following; copied from the Register of the Devon and Exeter Hospital, (in which, for some particular Reasons, warm bathing has not been much used) and allowing for the Difference of obstinate Cases sent, after trying all other Means to the Bath [Infirmary] for Relief.

Glass makes a distinction between palsies and paralytic disorders

Palsies admitted into the Devon and Exeter Hospital	104
Cured	40
Received great Benefit	28
Discharged for NonAttendance	4
Irregularity	1

At their own Request	5
As incurable	20
Dead	6
Paralytic Disorders admitted--	31
Cured	27
Received great Benefit	1
Discharged at their own Request	3

Adding both groups there was thus a cure/improvement rate of 71%. In John Summers' tract, where palsied and paralytic patients are not separated, he quotes the total number during the first nine years of the hospital's life:

Admitted	310
Cured	57
Much better	151
No better	45
Incurable	42
Dead	12
Remaining in house	3

This gives a cure/improvement rate of 67%; doubtless surprising and disappointing to such an advocate as Glass to find that the 'control' group did better than the treated group. A lesson for the careful selection of cases, indicating the risk of doing more harm than good, he was careful to state that some 'obstinate cases' were still sent from Exeter to Bath for relief. This was echoed by Andrew, who said, as Baker records:

> When the disease proves obstinate, we always endeavour to get our patients into the hospital at Bath; the Bath water, though not being a specific, being esteemed by us the most effectual remedy,both internally and externally used.

Richard Mead was also a well-known sceptic:

> And I have known some cases of paralytics, sent to Bath by a mistaken notion of their physicians, who upon coming out of the bath, were seized with a return of the apoplexy, which carried them off.[8]

This timely warning was acknowledged by Glass, who stressed the importance of adjustment of the body to different temperatures, and the avoidance of sudden change - the diehard conservative reiterating that this same track had been trodden by The Antients many centuries before. The purpose of the third bath being to prevent the danger of taking cold:

> contract the Pores and Vessels to their proper Dimensions, brace the Fibres, and give all Parts of the Body due Strength and Vigour.
> ... Upon the Whole then, the Operation of bathing was skilfully

contrived, cautiously managed, and happily applied by the antient Physicians, to purge the Vessels, Glands, and Receptacles from all useless, vitiated, or noxious Matter.

... to brace or relax the Fibres, as there was Occasion; to procure a free Passage for the Humours, and a proper Flow of them [thro' the several series of vessels]; in short, to answer, in most Cases, with the Assistance of Diet and Exercise, the principal Intentions of Cure, and reduce both Solids and Fluids to the most exact Standard of Perfect Health.

The phrase bracketed has been added to Thomas's copy by hand, presumably an afterthought. The concept of a series of vessels of decreasing size was essential to Boerhaave's theory of 'lentor' as a factor in disease, and Thomas Glass was a true Boerhaavian to the end.

Apart from spa towns, such as Bath, few provincial hospitals were as progressive as Exeter in the installation of a heated bath, or bagnio. The path had been laid down by St Thomas's Hospital in 1670, which ordered two stoves for the sweating of patients, who were undergoing treatment with mercury for the treatment of venereal disease; these were replaced in 1684 by a 'hot house', known later as the bagnio; this was fully described by William Boog Watson.[9] The reputation of the St Thomas's bagnio had spread to Edinburgh, and as the same author adds, when the Edinburgh Royal Infirmary of 1729, moved into a large new building in 1752, they resolved to incorporate a public bagnio for the benefit of the town; the model they chose was that at St Thomas's and a sketch plan of this installation was drawn up by John Hardie as an aid to the Edinburgh architect, John Adam.[10]

Echoes of Glass's enthusiasm for hot bathing still persisted into the nineteenth century. Dr John Blackall, that other great and beloved Exeter physician was equally convinced of their value. A patient of his, pleased with his treatment, said with somewhat ponderous facetiousness:

thank you most heartily, I hope the treatment may be successful, and having had the caldarium, the frigidarium, and the tepidarium, allow me to present you with the honorarium.[11]

Notes

(1)   Glass refers at this point to Dr William Oliver, *Essay on the Use and Abuse of warm bathing*, (Bath, 1791) p.18.

(2)   J. Delpratt Harris, *The Royal Devon and Exeter Hospital*, (Exeter, 1922), p.30.

(3)   The Bath Hospital was subsequently called The Mineral Water Hospital at Bath, and is now known as the Royal National Hospital for Rheumatic Diseases; see Roger Rolls, *The hospital of the nation : the story of spa medicine and the Mineral Water Hospital at Bath*, (Bath, 1988). John Summers was a physician at the Bath Hospital from 1748-1752.

(4)   William Musgrave, *De arthritide symptomatica dissertatio*, (Exeter, 1703). (Revised

edition Geneva, 1715) p.65.

(5)   John Huxham, *Observationes de aere et morbis epidemicus ab anno 1728-1748...accedit opusculum de morbo colico Damnoniensi,* (London, 1739-1752)

(6)   George Baker, 'An inquiry concerning the Endemial Colic of Devonshire', *The Medical Transactions of the College of Physicians,* (London, 1785), p. 175, having been read at the College June 29,1767.

(7)   R.M.S. McConaghey, 'Sir George Baker and the Devonshire Colic', *Medical History,* XI, (1967), pp. 345-360

(8)   Richard Mead, *The Medical Works of Richard Mead,* (Edinburgh, 1775), p.364.

(9)   William N. Boog Watson, 'The bagnio of St Thomas's Hospital', *Guy's Hospital Reports,* 121, 1972, pp. 199-204.

(10) John Adam was brother and partner of the better known Robert Adam.

(11) J. Delpratt Harris, op. cit. p.124.

CHAPTER XI
The Glass family

To establish Thomas Glass's origins as nearly as possible, it is necessary to reconcile information gleaned from the Devon Record Office with the account given in 1795 by Bartholemew Parr;[1] despite his envenomed value judgments, some credibility should be given to statements of fact, the source of which had been Thomas's surviving sister, Elizabeth, who died in 1800, as stated in an end note to Parr's Manuscript.

Parr stated that the family were dissenters, and that Michael, the great grandfather of Thomas, came from Aberdeen, in consequence of some religious and political disputes, about the beginning of the last century. He went on to say that he was in Tiverton as early as 1645, during the Civil War, that he was a dyer and brought his skill into the West Country, teaching the art to his son, Michael, and thence to his grandson. The earliest mention of a Glass at Tiverton was in 1603, when Elizabeth Glasse, wife of John, of Tiverton made an agreement to build on land on West Exe; they died respectively in 1635 and 1625. Their son, Peter, also a dyer, is named in a further lease in 1635, the date of his mother's death. He died in 1651.[2] In view of the location of the house on West Exe and the recent emergence of the name Glass at Tiverton, it is tempting to assume that Peter was the father of Thomas's great grandfather, Michael, though, if this is the case, it would seem to explode any link with Aberdeen. It is of course quite possible that the information provided by Elizabeth, Thomas's sister, was inaccurate and that the Aberdeen link, if there was one, applied to a member of an earlier generation. There is documentary evidence that Michael, who died in 1705, was the father of Thomas Glass, dyer, of West Exe, Thomas's grandfather, who died in 1736, four years after his grandson returned from Leyden.[3]

The Aberdeen link would seem to be even more of a red herring when one considers Michael's will; in it he left a small legacy to ten cousins, all of them with local names and with no reference to any Scottish kin. His mother was Mary Osmond, and her three nephews, Thomas, George and Peter are included with the other cousins.[4]

Thomas's mother was Elizabeth Handford, daughter of a respectable tanner of Calverley, near Tiverton. She had married his father, also Michael, on June 26, 1706; a substantial amount of property had been given to them on their marriage and consisted of:

> *The warehouse, with chamber, curtilage, stable and garden in West Exe, formerly part of a messuage held by John Way; messuage and land called The Coldharbour; two Fulling Mills and an old dwelling house and a close at Bolham, and dwelling houses built on a plot of ground in the Borough with the River Exe to the East.*[5]

A picture thus emerges of a prospering, Godfearing family, plying a skilled trade, and establishing itself, early in the eighteenth century.

Marriage to Mary Hodges may have brought Thomas four Daughters, but it also brought some problems in the shape of his mother-in-law, Lady Hodges, and to a lesser extent in that of George Hodges, Mary's brother. Mary's father, Sir Nathaniel, had left £1,500 to each of his daughters, to be paid to them as they married; in the marriage settlement Thomas had put land and property in the neighbourhood in trust for his wife, and Lady Hodges had added the £1,500, promising the trustees that the money would be paid over in six months time, when she herself had realised some other assets; in the mean time she was to pay interest on that sum.[6] In effect, after four years the money had still not been paid, despite repeated applications, and at the latter end of 1741 Thomas wrote to his mother-in-law in a mood of considerable exasperation:

> *Honoured Madam,*
> *I was very sorry to hear of brother George's illness and hope he is now in a fair way to recover.*
> *I have not a little reason to complain with regard to me and Polly.[7] When I married your daughter you had a thousand pounds in the bank, fifteen hundred in a mortgage of Mrs Stannyons, twelve hundred or more at Gravesend, so that there could no pretence be made for not paying of your bond till you had turned all you had into money. Far from that I was made to believe that I should have my wife's fortune in six months or thereabouts and it was on that very account that when Mr. Ambler made the bond for five per cent, I agreed to have it made for four.*
> *About a year afterwards I had a very fine opportunity of a mortgage of a thousand pounds and I desired you would pay me the money at a short warning which you complained of, but to make amends you promised to pay me four and a half per cent and that I should certainly be paid the whole when Mrs Stannyons mortgage was discharged. About a year since, when I desired you would pay me £500 some excuse or other was made of your inability to raise the money which gave me to distrust your management. When I desired to know, if you could not pay me, how Miss Hodges' fortune was to be paid, your answer was that she must trust as well as me. Now the money at the bank, that on Mrs. Stannyons mortgage, as well as that at Gravesend are all disposed of. Two younger children's fortunes are since paid and I must wait with patience till some houses which you can neither let nor sell are disposed of.[8]*
> *This is the just and fair treatment I have received from you. I am almost mad to think how tamely I have suffered myself to be abused, but will*

no longer delay redressing the injury done to me to the utmost of my power. Some time before Christmas I expect to be paid £500, or at that time shall draw a bill on you for that sum and after I am paid £500 insist you assign me the Sugar House as a security for paying me the remaining part of the bond, on which there will be due next February £1,297.[9]

There was no reply to this letter, so on August 30, Thomas wrote again, receiving a reply on behalf of his mother from George, on October 7, 1742. George's letters have, with one exception, a placatory tone, friendly to Thomas and affectionate towards his sister, Mary. He was himself a victim of his mother's feckless way with money, since a similar sum had been promised to him in respect of his own marriage to Polly; he also had had problems with his older brother, Nathaniel, also in debt, and to whom he too had lent money. George reviewed his mother's shaky financial situation, agreeing that she had made imprudent decisions, stating that Frances Dry, one of his two other sisters had not received her due on her marriage either:

as for money, it is absolutely out of her reach, and for want of it that you should use extreme measures with her, will by no means turn to account, for be assured, that if you should arrest her upon her bond, none of her friends will bail her and the consequence must be her going to jail, which will not at all sooner pay your debt, and as long as she is in being she must be maintained. The only advice I can give you in the affair is what I shall myself take, to wait with patience till she dies, and then we three youngest children must make the most we can of what she leaves behind her.

It seems that there was a prophetic element in this letter, for in February, 1744, Lady Hodges died; George wrote to Thomas with a copy of her will, a simple and rather pathetic matter:

Imprimis. To A. Middleton my best sable tippet agreable to my promise. Item. To M. Glass and F. Dry all my worldly apparrell and my great trunk of fine linnen to be equally divided between them, M. Glass taking my finest set of Damask Linnen as part of her share. Item. to M. Glass my silver tea kettle, lamp and stand. Item. To F. Dry my great silver saucepan and little silver coffee pot. Lastly that the Sugar House and lands at Topsham be disposed of as soon as conveniently may be and that the overplus, after Dr Glass is paid, to be equally divided between George Hodges and F. Dry, whom I appoint my Executors of this my last Will, requiring them to dispose of my household goods, rings and watch and plate not already mentioned for the payment of my just debts and funeral expenses.

George continued as follows:

The fifth part of the £2000 is now become yours and I think it will be prudent to dispose of it next month. I mean to sell the South Sea Annuities and divide the money which I hope will not produce less than £2000. It will be necessary for you to appear here (where shall be glad to see you) or appoint someone to act for you, to whom you must give Power of Attorney signed by your wife as well as yourself.

As to the Sugar House, we shall be glad you'll do your endeavour to dispose of it, and for the rest of the effects, I shall be glad to have your advice how to act....

The Sugar House deserves mention, not least because the building is still standing. It had passed to Lady Hodges (née Mary Buttall) from her relative Samuel Buttall, an importer of sugar from the West Indies, having purchased the building for his purposes in 1684. The raw sugar was brought to the port of Topsham in barrels, in the form of molasses, thence up the river by lighter, to be refined at the Sugar House and converted into sugarcones.[10]

It was more than twenty-five years before Thomas could sell the building, and only then after buying out the other interested parties. It was bought about 1770 by a Captain Robert Orme of the Coldstream Guards who built an imposing structure on the site, overlooking the beautiful Exe estuary, the river lapping the garden to the South and West. The name Sugar House remained until it was sold to Sir Alexander Hamilton, whose improving hand made many changes and who renamed it The Retreat. As with many such large mansions, it was later divided into flats; much of its thirty acres of grounds were sold for building, but its peace was disturbed for all time by the coming of the motorway, which strides across the Topsham road and the Exe estuary on giant legs, looking down on the elegant building of that other age with unselfconsciousness and no apology.

George Hodges continued to act for Thomas in connection with further investments, he wrote from Islington on September 22, 1762, and after some detailed comments about some stocks, he continued:

I think myself largely indebted for the trouble you have with my daughter, and I dont see how I shall make amends unless your whole family come to see us.

Mrs Hodges joins me in love to you and my sister and all the young folks.

Shortly after receiving this letter they were shocked to hear that George had died. Thomas wrote at once to George's son, Joseph:

Dear Nephew,

We are greatly affected with the unexpected account of your dear Father's death and feel the loss of a very near and esteemed relation and the distress the family are in on account of his death. This is the course of nature appointed for us by infinite Wisdom and Goodness and there-

138

fore without a doubt for the best ends which we cannot trace out as we cannot ascertain the immediate consequence of any one event. We don't doubt but that all of you will deserve your Mother's blessing by comforting her in the present desolate state and that you in particular will assist her to the utmost of your power in the management of her affairs.

No doubt it came as a considerable shock to both families to find that George died heavily in debt; his brother-in-law Middleton was already bankrupt, perhaps further unwitting victims, along with Nathaniel, of his mother's inept management of money. Of the £1,200 Thomas had asked George to invest for him, he only recovered one-third.

It had been in February 1762, that the Glass's eldest daughter, Mary, was married to John Vowler Parminter, an Exeter merchant.[11] Thus began a fruitful liaison betweeen the Glass and Parminter families and the delightful Miss Jane and Miss Mary Parminter, beacons of eighteenth century eccentricity. Of these Jane was the eldest, born in 1747 at Lisbon, where her father, John, had a wine exporting business; Mary was the daughter of Richard Parminter, John's nephew, and Mary Walrond, so they were one generation apart, second cousins, rather than first cousins as is often stated. In 1784 they set off on the Grand Tour for a period of ten years along with Elizabeth, Jane's invalid sister, and a friend, Miss Colville, keeping a journal about their adventures.[12] On their return, Jane and Mary built a truly remarkable house near Exmouth; this was a sixteen sided building, in effect round, overlooking the estuary of the River Exe; positioned, it is said, so that they would be the first to see the invading armies of Napoleon, being sure that this would be the avenue of his attack. Every room had two doors so that should the French soldiers take

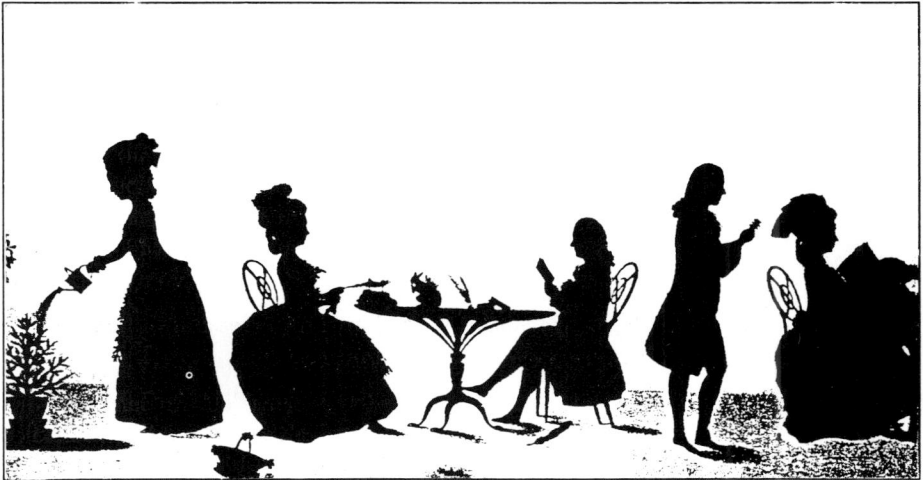

The Parminters at home, 1783, by Francis Torond (reproduced by kind permission of the National Trust).

them by surprise they could elude them by moving from one room to another, closing sliding doors behind them and so escape. The house is also remarkable in that it is the repository of an enormous collection of eighteenth century bricabrac, amassed on their grand tour, much of it, particularly feathers and shells, used for interior decoration in a bizarre and curiously attractive way, something that took many years. It is called A la Ronde.[13]

John Vowler Parminter was the brother of Richard, Mary's father, and his six children were thus first cousins to Mary of A La Ronde. She and Jane were early feminists; to the east of the house they built a small chapel, a school and some almshouses: the school for female children only and the almshouses for elderly spinsters. Mary Parminter's will required that the house should be occupied only by unmarried kinswomen. The very name of the house is enigmatic; Jane's mother's maiden name was Arboin, Mary's mother's was Walrond. One may speculate that there is a deeper significance beyond the virtually circular shape of the house.

Ann, the third daughter of Thomas and Mary Glass, was married in April 1778 to John Lowder, a banker of Southampton,[14] they settled in Bath, and they too had six children, one of whom, John Lowder junior, was a well-known architect. There is some dispute as to how much of the design of A la Ronde was attributable to Jane Parminter herself and how much to John Lowder. His Bath and District National School of 1816 was circular in form, with wedge-shaped classrooms; he was thus both a first cousin of Mary Parminter and a grandson of Thomas Glass.

In 1762, the year of the marriage of Mary Glass and John Vowler Parminter, Benjamin Heath and his wife left Bedford House for Teignmouth and the Glass's move to Bartholemew Yard cannot have occurred much after that; for when the house was demolished in 1773 it had been empty for a considerable time, to be redeveloped as the elegant Bedford Circus by the builders Stribling and Painter.

The only one of the four Glass daughters who did not marry was Elizabeth, who died at the early age of 38. Was it Elizabeth to whom Bartholemew Parr darkly referred?

> *this external prosperity was sullied by domestic calamities, by calamities attributed to himself. He has been accused of a stern churlishness and inattention to the tenderest wishes of his daughters and of occasioning all the dreadful consequences of their disappointment. This accusation I know to be false ...*

Was this, perhaps, one of the warts for which we have long been seeking, along with a mercenary streak directed at his mother-in-law? Or was it another sly daub, from which Parr hastened too quickly to dissociate himself?

The youngest daughter, Melony (also known as Melina or Melanie), married Samuel Daniell, a banker of Yeovil in November 1777. There were no children of this marriage. Samuel was the brother of Dr George Daniell (1760-1822), the physician to the Devon and Exeter Hospital who inaugurated the medical library there in 1813, and which for a long time sequestrated Thomas Glass's books, specifically bequeathed to Exeter Cathedral.

Conclusion

> *Pygmies are pygmies still, though perched on Alps;*
> *And pyramids are pyramids in vales.*
> *Each man makes his own stature, builds himself:*
> *Virtue alone outbuilds the Pyramids;*
> *Her monuments shall last when Egypt's fall.*
> EDWARD YOUNG, *Night vi*

Eighteenth Century morbidity being what it was, it was not surprising that Thomas Glass's final years should be clouded with the sadness of bereavement. He had outlived his brothers; Peter having died in 1758 at the age of 36, Samuel in 1773, and Michael in 1781. Elizabeth, his second and unmarried daughter, died in 1780. When Mary Parminter the oldest daughter died in 1776, the Glass household was augmented by six grandchildren who were largely cared for by Mary Wills, the Glass daughters' old family nurse. This arrangement also was attended by tragedy, for the only grandson died, aged 15, in 1783. Mary's husband, John Vowler Parminter, remarried.

Without doubt, however, the most severe blow was the death of his wife in 1783; as Parr has it: 'of an asthma, a disease which his skill could not cure and which it could not always alleviate'. In a moment of uncharacteristic gentleness, Parr had described her as 'the woman whom he had never ceased to love with unabating tenderness'.

Thomas's own health began to break down soon afterward; though long retired from the hospital, his former colleagues paid him the honour of electing him President of the hospital in March, 1785; the only occasion that a member of the honorary staff was ever given this accolade. He was not however able to complete his Presidential year, and he died on February 5, 1786, having suffered for a long time from a painful and disagreeable condition of the urinary organs.

The *Exeter Flying Post*, child of the redoubtable bookseller, Robert Trewman, printed a fairly predictable obituary on February 9:

> *On Sunday last, died in the 77th year of his age, after a long and painful illness, the celebrated Dr Thomas Glass, whose extensive and successful practice had for many years deservedly placed him at the head of his profession: nor was he less valuable in his private capacity than eminent in his public station, not confining within the limits of*

*his profession only his assistance to the necessitous, but relieving their
wants by various other acts of liberality; thus happily uniting the characters of a Great Physician and a Good Man.*

To Jenkins, twenty years later, the aura was still apparent; writing of St.
David's church:

*In an obscure corner of the yard, behind the church, is interred the body
of the late Dr Glass of Exeter, whose professional skill, eminent
learning, and amiable disposition, justly acquired the esteem of all his
numerous acquaintance.*[15]

The grave is near the southwest gate, together with those of his wife and four
daughters, Elizabeth Glass, Mary Parminter, Anne Lowder and Mellony
Daniel.

It is perhaps of significance that three of his four trustees were apothecaries,
William Pitfield, William Luscombe, and John Codrington; the fourth was the
Reverend Robert Tarrant. To each he left a sum of £50 to buy a piece of plate
'or any other thing they may think proper'.[16]

Each of his servants was left £10, and Mary Wills, the elder, 'who has served
me and my family during the best part of her Life', was in addition left an
annuity of £10 per annum. 'If more should be wanted to supply her with the
Necessaries of Life in her helpless age my Daughters and GrandDaughters
will remember the Care their Maid took of them in their Infancy and
Childhood.' Mary Wills was also remembered by Thomas's sister, Elizabeth,
in her will of 1791:[17]

*I give to the Dean and Chapter of the Cathedral Church of Exeter all my
medical printed Books on condition they will assign them a place in
their Library, order the titles of them to be inserted in their Catalogue,
and permit any Physician being an Inhabitant of the City of Exeter to
have recourse to them at proper times in the library ...*

The collection of books has remained intact, its historical value has been
immeasurably enhanced by the feet of the years, and it is a fitting memorial
to its originator.

As a final small gesture to the medical fraternity, he gave a mourning ring
to every physician, surgeon, and apothecary in the city or suburbs of Exeter.

The greater part of his will was directed at his two remaining daughters, his
grandchildren, and his sisters, Mary and Elizabeth, still living at Tiverton. He
left £50 to the poor of Tiverton, to be distributed at the discretion of his sisters;
he had already, in 1782, given five dwelling houses in Water Lane, Tiverton,
for the support of the minister of the Baptist congregation in Tiverton.[18]

As to the poor of Exeter, he executed three deeds poll of £50 each, upon the
Exeter Turnpike, in favour of the Minister of St Mary Arches, the interest
thereof to be employed in teaching poor children of St Mary Arches, St

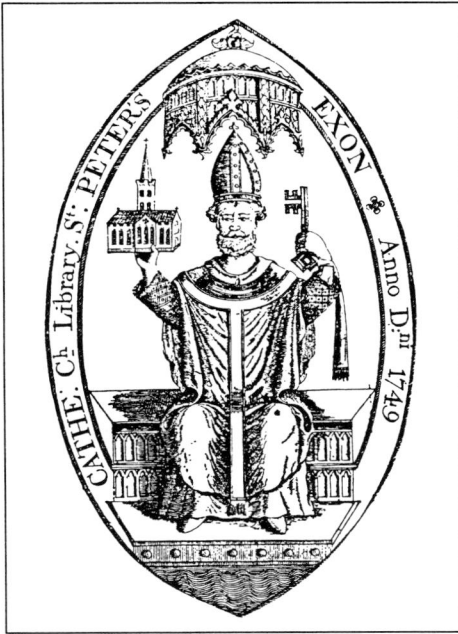

Bookplate, Exeter Cathedral Library, 1749.

Olave's, and Allhallows on the Walls the boys to read and the girls to read and work at the needle.

Thomas Glass's mark on his own and succeeding generations was fourfold; his written work, both published and unpublished, his library, still enjoyed today, his bloodline, and the warm feelings he engendered in his patients and colleagues, which echoed down the corridors of Exeter for another fifty or sixty years.

There was of course the discordant voice of Bartholemew Parr, who depicted him as something of an ogre, and as having achieved his reputation by good fortune and by using the efforts and talents of others. He was not in his view much of a Latin scholar and clung too doggedly to the outmoded beliefs of Boerhaave. There was some dark family secret, he had shown himself on occasion to be uncaring, and his general persona was harsh and unfriendly. Articulate commentators, such as Downman, Polwhele, Jenkins, Oliver, and Munk did not seem to share this opinion.[19] At the bar of history, Parr reveals himself to be full of bitterness and uncharity.

Notes

(1)   Bartholemew Parr, *Biographical Anecdotes of the late Dr Glass of Exeter*, (1795), MS, Library of the Royal College of Physicians of London.

(2)   DRO, Reference 257 M T 113128.

(3)   DRO, Reference 49/9/6/ 190214.

(4)   DRO, Reference 49/9/6/ 211a.

(5)   DRO, Reference 49/9/6/ 195.

(6)   DRO, Reference 49/9/6/ 210.

(7)   Polly was George Hodges's wife. A similar sum had been promised by Lady Hodges at Polly's marriage.

(8)   Mary's sisters were Frances Dry and Ann Middleton.

(9)   DRO, Reference 72/1/2/ 1. Glass's correspondence with Lady Hodges. George Hodges and other family members are all included in this reference (quoted by permission of the Devon and Exeter Institution),

(10) DRO, Reference DD 100260, deeds of the Sugar House.

(11) DRO, Reference 49/9/6/213

(12) Unfortunately all but the first part of the journal is lost, see account by the Reverend Oswald Reichel, *Transactions of the Devonshire Association*, Vol. 34 (1902), pp 265-275.

(13) A la Ronde, near Exmouth is now the property of the National Trust.

(14) DRO, Reference 49/9/6/ 214.

(15) Alexander Jenkins, *History and Description of the City of Exeter*, (Exeter,1806), p.354.

(16) DRO, Reference 2309 B/W 111 b (quoted by permission of Messrs Crosse, Wyatt, Verney and Ayre, solicitors).

(17) DRO, Reference 2309 B/W 110/12.

(18) W. Harding, *History of Tiverton*,(Tiverton 1845), Vol. 2, p. 253.

(19) H. Downman, *Poems to Thespia*, (Exeter, 1792)
R. Polwhele, The History of Cornwall, (London 1806), vol VII p.128.
G. Oliver (alias Curiosus), *Biographies of Eminent Exonians* (newspaper cuttings) in Devon and Exeter Institution.
W. Munk, *Western Times,* 1855, 13 Oct. p.8.

Appendix

Translation from the Latin of the Inaugural Dissertation submitted by Thomas Glass for the degree of MD at the University of Leyden, July 13, 1731.

Atrophy in general, Phthisis of the Lungs, and those Particular Diseases, which lead to it.

The whole human body consists of both solid and fluid parts; all solid parts, of any kind, arise from the fluid, except a very small particle found in the primary egg and called the carina [rudimentary spine].[1] [In the fowl] it may be shown that this, made from egg albumen, with only the extra influence of incubation, hatches out as a chick in the space of three weeks. Ruysch has shown that Man is formed from a similar such carina, floating in an almost identical humour, enclosed in a special membrane (ensuring the stability of the whole structure).

It is clear that nutrition and growth are not brought about by external influence; everything in the egg is made from albumen, causing the carina to grow by a defined force in each dimension, not uniformly, but clearly according to method and rule; at the same time such new material is provided as is suitable for the laying down of the solid parts. By analogy it may be shown that the same happens at the inception of a human being, and by this process the Foetus grows into a perfect Adult.

That this may be achieved, continual addition of new material is absolutely vital, impossible unless the humours can permeate every single part of the body. It follows that both the body of the carina and of adult man must be composed of minute pores or canals. infinitely small, as far as one can tell: a doctrine often confirmed by experiment.

Egg albumen, before it can be made suitable for the nourishment of the embryo, needs to undergo a great deal of dissolution and thinning. Bellini has demonstrated visually that this happens by the process of incubation mentioned; however the subtlety of this is better understood by reason; consider both the texture of the amnion and the amazingly fine nature of the carina's vessels which must let this substance permeate and flow through them to give nutrition. If the carina has as many vessels and they are as convoluted as in the perfect foetus, one cannot fail to recognise its infinite delicacy; even so it is readily credible, seeing that man's development from foetus to full stature is a continual process; and all the while, it is believed, no new vessels are created; on the contrary, anatomy and injections have shown that very many are actually destroyed.[2]

From this subtle humour, able to flow through the vessels of the carina, minute particles may be formed, which grow and coalesce, and on by increasing steps to particles of the largest size. Thus from these beginnings all firm parts are laid down; their diverse form arising from the complex arrangement of these structures.

There are many great workers in the field of detailed anatomy, Malpighi, Leeuenhoek, Hook, and Ruysch; over a long period they have taught, with the aid of injections and microscopy, that large vessels arise from small, fibres from fibrils, large bones from small, and so on, always ascending this road by small steps from the minuscule to the infinitely large. Certainly they have been unable to achieve a complete explanation, only in such elusive terms as defy full understanding. Thus by this method of nutrition and the resolution of the adult body into its fundamental parts, it may be stated that man is made from this primitive humour, by no means a delicate substance, by its perfusion through the smallest vessels.

In all these activities associated with nutrition, on which the preservation of life and health depends, minute particles, only weakly adherent, are rubbed off by the fluids set in motion by the force of the heart and arteries; these join together again elsewhere, where they regain that cohesive property which they have lost. If they are not properly attached they are not able to develop into solid structures, so resulting in a useless mass of tissue, eliminated from the body at an early stage through its natural channels. The vessels, in fact, become worn down and thinned by the humours constantly pouring through them, and no longer able to contain them, leakage occurs through the sides of the smallest. On the other hand humours may lose their natural soothing nature and become so acrid that they interfere with nutrition; acrimonies may soon weigh down the whole body, unless help is at hand from elsewhere. Those who have died of starvation provide examples of this; thus the living body may destroy itself in a short space of time unless there is daily replacement of all tissue lost. The damaged area needs to be filled with particles similar to those lost, by the application of whatever influence is necessary. These particles are thus produced from that same fluid from which they were originally created, that is the egg albumen. That internal humour, to be sure, derived so recently from the blood, follows almost the same path as when the organs and vessels of the fowl are first laid down, incubated by warmth, dispersed through its substance, and elaborated; whatever thereafter is received by the vessels of the carina is further refashioned; eventually becoming by proper application what is needed for nourishment and development of the fowl.

Food, drink, and air are ideal material for the healthy body, for its various functions, and for making blood, the source of serum; as with albumen and the egg, it seems that there is a wide gulf between nutrition and its source.

Nevertheless, because natural needs dictate it, as one learns from books of Physiology (to be closely scrutinised), there needs also to be respite from life's heavy burden.

The humour then is so refined that it passes through the smallest pores, especially rich in those particles previously eroded by wear and tear, and most fitted for restoration, requiring only the application of the necessary influence. This, the ultimate, most elaborate, and natural process may with justice may be called true nutrition.

On this premise I can now discuss the Greek word ATROPHY

('α' privative, 'τροφη' nutrition), one may interpret it as defective nourishment, whatever the cause. Atrophy means for me, therefore, that state of the body, where whatever is worn away by the action of the body, is not replaced by firm parts.

Diagnosis rests on total weakening of the body, by distortion of almost every function, and by emaciation of the whole exterior aspect. The exception is where humours stagnate in the vessels, which become distended, increasing evenly the shapeless outline of the body; Leucophlegmasia and Dropsy provide examples; nor will those who understand nutrition be surprised that it is a very different matter from being overfilled with fluid.

The immediate causes of the disease are known: a fault in the nutrifying humour, or its lack, or finally the failure of the necessary application. The fault in nutrient humour arises either because insufficient is produced by concoction of foods, or conversion of them to our true nature, by alteration of healthy humours, or because they have become alien and corrupt.

Coction is impeded if foods ingested are by their nature too tough to be properly softened and changed by the body's powers, thus the fault here is in the substance ingested, with which the body, however sound, cannot deal.[3] These are what Celsus calls useless foods. This happens in an already weakened body, with some defect, due to fault in one or more natural functions, especially bad coction in the first passages, loss of lung function, or excessive weakness of all vessels.[4]

Almost all humours of the body are made from chyle alone, its corruption makes them likewise corrupt; because this happens in various ways so Cacochymia also has various origins.[5] Food eaten and improperly digested retains its own properties, only undergoing change in the first passages that would have occurred if kept outside the body in the same degree of warmth and humidity; this change is known as spontaneous corruption; chemists have shown us that foods putrefy of their own accord, some becoming sour, others glutinous and malodorous; besides doing all kinds of harm to the humours.

The intrinsic quality of every Cacochymia must be sedulously investigated, an easy matter for the skilled physician, from existing and continuing signs, and so countered by the requisite remedies.

Since it is a fact that a happy digestion encourages Euchymia, a few general rules of diet may help, without being burdensome. Not everybody concocts all foods equally, but each concocts those suited to his nature, taking into account his normal disposition. Food is concocted best and quickest by people who have vital energy and great bodily strength; those of a feeble and chilly constitution concoct slowly and with difficulty, the one tending towards acidity, the other to putrescence. If an excessive amount is eaten, or it is undercooked, good chyle is not made; the first results in acridity and putrescence, the other in insufficient assimilation.

Probably changes to ingested food occur in a shorter time with stronger digestive powers, but weaker digestions take longer, because of differing temperaments; thus tougher foods for strong, robust men, being hard, do not tend to putrescence and are not very stimulating, with these water is the most suitable drink; to such people eupeptic and easily putrescent foods are harmful: these are only well-digested by the weak, the cold and slothful, and with these a stimulating drink is beneficial. It is known that all food is suitable for either type, if welldigested; moderate amounts allay hunger and thirst, so the body has enough to sustain it for a time and accordingly abstains from more. Nourishment of humours is necessary to oppose any morbid tendency, often shown by immediate awakening of appetite; so nature demands what kind of food the body requires, as long as no harm results, although it may seem absurd or contrary to the strict rules of the art. A gradual transition must be made from one kind of food to another, especially if they are intrinsically of different natures; unaccustomed foods are concocted least well, so one must either augment or decrease a little at a time; however good the food, it is important to add that it is not well-digested when taken in large amounts.

In summer, foods tend to be thin and humid, in winter hard and dry, striking a mean at other times; this rule may be modified according to whether the district is hot or cold. If at a single meal a less than robust person eats tough food, then what is more easily digested, then easier still, coction will be bad; if the reverse process occurs it will be good. Galen first told us this and Bennet confirmed it by experiment. Hypochondriacs and the less robust have poor digestions. Quality of life for phlegmatic and inactive people depends on the small intestine; except where due to disease a good appetite promises a happy digestion. Tightness and pressure on the belly, dullness of body and mind go with belching and an unpleasant taste; regurgitation of food, nausea, discomfort, sometimes headache and anxiety about food are all signs of faulty coction; fortunately these things are normally absent where there is levity and liveliness of mind. Too much chyle causes a crude admixture with the blood four to six hours after eating, resulting in slight fever, difficult breathing and often cough.

Enough has been said about coction in the first passages; the chyle requires assistance in its formation, but it is still a foreign substance, needing complete assimilation into man's nature, just as the forces which weaken, constrain and mould the body before it is complete; these are in fact derived from the vital actions of the heart, vessels, and good blood; meantime heterogeneous substances unsuitable for assimilation are eliminated by convenient channels to the outside. Where circulation of humours flags or a sufficient quantity of good blood is not at hand, needed assimilation will always be lacking. Young leisured people provide examples of this, especially young girls and the elderly, and those who have lost a great deal of blood, even though the body was completely robust beforehand. In all these cases watery, pituitous humours may build up a defect in the vessels because of attrition &c.

Thus it becomes clear that the greatest demand for assimilated material is in the lungs; for here actions of vessels on humours, and reciprocally humours on vessels, and one humour on another are greatest: for no drop of humour enters the aorta which has not beforehand passed through the lungs: there is a certain time needed therefore for passage through the lungs and a certain time for the rest of the body; since all types of vessel in the whole body far outnumbers those in the lung, the flow of humours there must be more rapid; speed greatly increases attrition, so this will be much greater in the lung than in all the rest of the body; but the unique nature of the vessels of the lung and the particular act of respiration increases this attrition to an amazing extent, as the lung vessels vary continually in shape and size and at the same time are squeezed most vigorously; while from one part the force of air presses as if rushing into a vacuum, from another there is resistance as the pressure is overcome by the organs of expiration.

Further it should be understood that as many kinds of vessel occupy a single lung as occupy the whole body; for the reason that every kind of humour must flow through them, and neither injections nor anatomy have anywhere revealed that they contain anything more refined; but if vessels of all types are intertwined there will also be humours of all kinds derived from them for the use of the whole body. So it is very clear with what great care blood is fashioned, first from chyle, then from nutrient juices, and how the correct formation of humours requires healthy lungs; nevertheless they are subject to many perils; the weakest point is the fabric which constantly withstands an unbelievable strain. Since crude chyle is forced initially through the smaller vessels it results only in viscosity and acridity; what obstructions and harm will this not produce? For every humour, viscous or sharp, likely to block the circulation, corrupted by stagnation or insinuated from outside, may taint the body; whence it is not surprising that damage to the lung may be a very frequent cause of Atrophy.

149

Healthy humours may change into unhealthy ones; or the fluids may undergo some harmful change within themselves; already it has been stated that humours may cause damage to the circulation, already depressed; indeed because of this they must be expelled through the cleansing passages of the body, for otherwise if retained they would cause injury.

So it is apparent that great harm occurs from day to day blocking of the Sanctorian perspiration, the urine, or certain other customary evacuations[6]. And it is a fact that both humours and hectic fevers distort an excessive circulation, frequently leading to continuals and intermittents, or an imperfect cure.

All humours, healthy or morbid, found in the body, stagnating in that degree of heat necessary to life and even more to health, may become corrupted and acrid; to a large extent they become putrescent. Such corruption anywhere in the body invades its surroundings, spreading like fire to the blood through dried up veins. This is the source of many hectic fevers, differing only in the location of the trouble. Plethora, always an unhealthy state whatever the origin, brings about stagnation of humours, a known source of trouble; thereafter other ills may befall where there is faulty assimilation of unaccustomed foods, due to a slowing of essential movement of humours. Miasma in the air or perhaps different food eaten in areas where Tabes[7] is an endemic disease, seemingly corrupts the humours; so various poisons, whether taken daily or only once, have produced languid Atrophy. Which kind of blood is corrupted by bile I do not know, for it is not yet agreed that the biliary circulation joins that of the blood.

Deprivation of nutrient humour may occur, the second cause of atrophy; for example, with poor blood flow chyle may not receive its lost replenishments, or the body may be afflicted by constant heavy loss of humours. In the first instance there may be an abundance of chyle even though scanty in the first passages; this can occur from lack of food; it may be that sufficient is made but not passed onwards, or it is consumed by worms, or paths that give access to the blood are blocked: a complete fistula of intestines may have been made by invading ulcers, or the openings of the lacteals are blocked, or there may be a stubborn scirrhus of mesenteric glands or tumour at the root of the mesentery, as dissection of wasted people has shown; many obstacles of this sort have a profound effect. The thoracic duct, also supplied with blood vessels, may become inflamed, suppurate and become eroded. It may also happen that there is too great a flood of humours through and beyond the normal channels.

Atrophy is commonly seen at the French court, where it is customary to chew sweetsmelling lozenges, so causing copious loss of saliva; prolonged nursing, Diabetes, excessive purging, Fluor albus, nonvirulent Gonorrhea, over-indulgence in sexual matters (here Tabes dorsalis may be mentioned), excessive sweating, and frequent vomiting are all possible causes; one could add profuse oozing from large ulcers, or repeated bleeding from the nose or elsewhere. Such manifestations frequently lead to Tabes. Finally none will doubt that the body may become exhausted for any of these minor reasons, and as a result may fail to gain nourishment.

The last cause of Atrophy which must be mentioned (namely a failure of the necessary application), arises from the expenditure of energy or, amounting to the same thing, either a very torpid circulation or a very violent one; this happens with continual Fevers, which if recurring often, over a long time, lead to Marasmus: in every case of Atrophy the main features are weakened pulse and loss of flesh, mainly at some distance from the heart, first noticeable in fact in the legs; this state cannot last long without harming humours. Further, the necessary application of the nutrient humours is blocked by damage to vessels through which they flow; thus laxity, rigidity, narrowing, obstruction and loss can arise, and being ultimately the cause of rigidity developing in the smallest vessels, I see them as the particular cause of Marasmus and Death in the elderly: even though humours may be carried back through arteries, veins, or larger nerves, flow is blocked or diverted for some reason; in this way Atrophy arises in those regions which they subserve.

Hippocrates observed a complete Tabes from injury to the spinal medulla: possible when the medulla is filling with blood, for if its blood vessels are too greatly distended it is almost certain that adjoining parts will be compressed.
Such disease may arise from excessive amount of blood in the whole body, by failure to limit the amount of blood made or because egress through the spinal veins is blocked. The same illness may occur from the venae cavae (as distinct from the spinal medulla) when distended with catarrh, dropsical fluid or bile. Another form of Tabes may occur from flow into the medulla, an obstruction to the medullary vessels, erosion of them, or an effusion of fluid between medullary membranes. Thus the medulla is itself compressed and, if this persists, corrupted. The medulla spinalis may eventually dry out because of blockage in the venules of the medulla (these are arteries which carry blood to the medullary cortex, for the secretion of the succus nervosus), or else when for some reason the doorway from brain to medulla has been obstructed.

Lastly I believe that Atrophy may easily arise in this way in all parts of the body. I have set out its causes comprehensively; they are often combined.
It is not possible to give an all-embracing Prognosis, this must be sought from known causes and the nature of the illness present.
Indications of cure are such that a specific revealed cause is removed if

possible, and the disease dealt with by remedies contrary to its nature. Strictly it would be necessary to describe all diseases arising from a defect of nutrition and also report the precise cure of each, so much at variance with the normal starting point and goal of Academic practice: one point however I would stress to my utmost, is that Phthisis of the lungs provides an opportunity for lengthy discussion of a number of such matters.

Pulmonary PHTHISIS is decay of the whole body arising from ulcer in the lung, due largely to preceding inborn disease. Experience has shown that an ulcer is formed as follows: from Distillation[8] of acrid fluid into the lungs, by pulmonary vessels becoming clogged with crude and viscous humour, putrefying there; from Haemoptysis; from unresolved Inflammation of the lungs, and finally from thoracic Empyema.

On Inflammation of the lungs and thoracic Empyema I have nothing to say; the history and cure of these are to be sought in the writings of renowned Physicians, such as the Aphorisms of Boerhaave, who gathered the true wisdom of the Antients, and set it all out in an orderly manner, (unlike the observations of the Moderns): most importantly this same sedulous servant of nature has revealed the most secret purposes of his mistress, treading in her footsteps, and evolving a true and stable doctrine to the huge reward of the human race.

Because, it may be said, other diseases mentioned are often a starting point for Phthisis and frequently combined with it, I have thought it necessary to discuss these to give forewarning of the approach of Phthisis, which, once established, is difficult to heal; without this foundation it is scarcely possible to establish a cure.

Of the acrid Catarrh

Catarrh, from the Greek καταρρευς, indicates a downward flow of a certain humour from one part to another; particularly from the head to areas below it; however modern thinking refutes this doctrine. By acrid Catarrh I mean the deposition of acrid humour in lungs and bronchi, together with the cough thus produced.

Diagnosis is easily grasped, Hippocrates described it thus: at the commencement, slight fever and rigor, chest and back affected; there is also troublesome cough, sometimes painful, with expectoration of much salty saliva. This makes Distillation much heavier, with salty bloodstained sputum, expelled immediately on waking in the morning and four, five, or six hours after food, by coughing or hawking; this will be mentioned when I come to Haemoptysis.

The immediate factor seems to be a separation of the acrid and foreign humour in bronchial or pulmonary vessels, which nature endeavours to excrete through these passages; the effect of this, mainly the acrimony, on the sensitive bronchial membrane is to excite a tickling cough. Very often a severe cough accompanies this distillation; this is because the humour is thin, and settling down on the little vesicles or minor vessels of the bronchi, is expelled upwards into the larger vessels by coughing; there it is so thin that it is dispersed alongside them, the pressure causing great irritation of the nerves.

So the main cause of the disease may be stated thus: anything that sets up acridity of the blood, making acrid material spread to the lungs; I have listed various ways in which acrimony of the blood may occur, but there is no more frequent cause of Catarrh than that which arises from obstruction of the Sanctorian perspiration.

I believe the skin to be the proper organ for evacuating very acrid and subtle humours, conveyed by the circulation and prone to putrefaction. If its more important functions are not fulfilled, the onset of problems will soon testify to the defect: besides this everyday function, an exit is often provided for humours shed during a continual fever, thus already almost putrefying; so the living body, although reeling, is restored to health. But, as often happens, if the way through the skin is denied, the humour whose function is to make perspiration, floods the lungs. It is evident, for example, that the pores of the skin are frequently closed by cold.

Is it necessary to attempt to demonstrate that nature in trying to free itself from foreign matter, often does so by separating it from healthy humours, forcing it this way or that and finally evacuating it? Or isn't this more than satisfactorily explained by the manifold critical abscesses of febrile matter as shown by Venereal Ulcers? What else do Podagra, very offensive seasonal diarrhoea, and numerous other conditions known well to Physicians show us? A head cold or minor complaint which often precedes a feverish Catarrh may bear witness to the way nature attempts to remove diseased matter; this opinion is largely confirmed by the crossflow of acrid humours from the lungs to other parts, thus freeing them; on the other hand, the flow may be seen to go from elsewhere to the lung. Bennet, whose teaching I strive to the utmost to follow in this essay, gives many examples of this.

The reason for the deposition of acrimony of the blood in the lungs is largely hidden from us, but it may be related in some way to the true nature of the materials concerned; thus we may see the humours affected by scammony deposited in the bowel, by mercury in the mouth &c; whatever impedes free circulation of the humours through the extremities or the surface of the body is more likely to do this: stopping the blood flow through a limb and obstruction of its arteries both make it cold.

Malformation of the lungs is another factor, recognised by a flat and narrow chest, winged scapulae, and breathlessness on slight movement; this deformity is caused by progressive disease, particularly in those disposed to it; thus in Phthisis all acridity rushes to the lungs causing excessive laxity and weakness of the pulmonary vessels, compared with the rest of the body; finally, as Hippocrates has stated, every part draws to itself whatever is hot and uncomfortable; it is possible that cough is related to this.

Prognosis may be determined once the nature of the acrimony is established, and the existing conditions, together with the state of the lung. It could be that the acrimony at the time is so fixed in the blood that removal is impossible, even with difficulty, because the cause cannot be removed; or suppose Catarrh is profuse, frequent, longlasting and very acrid; or the lung is malformed and inherently weak, especially with progressive Catarrh, to which it is prone; where symptoms of disease increase daily; particularly acute cough, even more when intermittent, in morning or afternoon, with slight breathlesness and sense of pressure on the chest; all these in a patient with a delicate nature and slender build where the body wastes day by day from progressive disease, would be reasons to fear Phthisis, on account of the smallest vessels interwoven in the bronchial membrane. Here particularly, the vesicles of Malpighi may be eroded by acrid humour or so macerated in it, that they are prey to easy dissolution, completed eventually by violent shaking and straining coughs. From all aspects it is possible to see how an ulcer of the lung can arise which, for all these reasons, enlarges day by day; alternatively the whole fabric of the lung may dissolve, producing foully offensive sputum.

Hippocrates described the wasting caused by this disease: in its progress, he said, the body becomes thin, all except the legs; these swell, however, with contraction of feet and nails; from the shoulder down the arms become thin and weak. The throat looks as if covered with wool and the breath whistles as if through a reed, the dryness lasting as long as the disease; the body is intensely weak; anyone in this state perishes, broken down, within the year.

Haemoptysis may also occur, either from minute vessels, purely serous, or from exhalant vessels, so disposed that they already transmit more than the normal amount of red blood, aided in this by cough; then, very often, acrid bloody sputum may be expelled at certain times, that produced first overcoming other acrimonies. This tendency of minor vessels to remove red blood is very common in the body: the menstrual flow, the bloody stools of persistent diarrhoea, the extraordinary haemorrhages of scurvy and many other examples are sufficient demonstration of this. Moreover Haemorrhage still occurs as a result of an erosion, especially where mucus fails to seal the bronchus; thin people are often prone to this risk, where there is a constant dripping moisture, or eventually the violence of coughing ruptures the vessels.

A lesser acrimony introduced into the blood for some minor reason is easily overcome; for example, the perspiration may have been blocked by an external agent, such as cold; here, if the lungs are wellformed and healthy,

154

nature alone, perhaps with minimal support, may rapidly prevail.

Curative indications are: to remove and evacuate the oppressive humour from the lungs through other passages of the body, so that the acrimony affecting the blood is overcome and the cause is removed; finally, help must be brought to the lungs themselves.

If it is known that an acrid humour, trickling into the lungs, is normally evacuated through other channels, it must be diverted as nearly as possible through the same passages. A Revulsion in general comes from increasing the flow of humours at the proper site.[9] This may diminish the resistance of vessels here, affecting the whole body, bringing warmth and pain to the part treated and, if sluggish, stimulating circulation. Where it is plain that all humours abound in acrimony, which nature is trying to drive through the lungs, if possible an easier safer way must be prepared, isolating and finally expelling the acrid humour: nevertheless nature cannot be forced to do this, it is only possible to open those channels through which, as experience shows, such humours are usually evacuated.

I will state briefly those methods approved by the authorities. Bennet recommends issues[10] cut sufficiently deeply into those places where the body sweats automatically and freely; blistering agents may likewise be applied. The openings of vessels of Schneider's membrane maybe relaxed and opened; this is often the seat of Catarrh and is in harmony with tissue clothing the bronchi. Here emollient decoctions, may be used or tepid milk diluted with water, drawn through the nostrils from the cupped hand at frequent intervals; or gargled or swallowed, relaxing the vessels of the throat, oesophagus &c .

Also, there is a natural tendency to expel almost any unhealthy substance through the intestine, provoking Diarrhoea which forces nature to take this path, a source of satisfaction to the physician; therefore this channel must be opened, by relaxing the vessels of the intestines and provoking a mild looseness. Remedies found satisfactory are decoct. prunorum, or stewed prunes, cassia, tamarind, manna, sal. polycrest., tartarus, rob. sambuc;[11] other than this there is the mild laxative made from flour, wellknown to physicians, which given as a drink is happily accepted by the patient; as much as the stomach can take, three or four times a day, and repeated often.

These seem to me to follow the practise of Hippocrates, who in the same disease gave boiled asses' milk or cow's milk or that of the goat, to the point of light purgation. If there is no yielding to this, it must be ensured that a strong body is stirred up more forcibly, which Hippocrates never doubted would follow a strong emetic and sharp purge; he was accustomed to purge only four times a year, twice upwards, twice downwards. Acrid material flowing to the intestine and then rising to the lungs must be controlled only by purgatives, of particular use when perspiration is prevented by cold air.

Diuretics also, if not heat producing, sometimes have their uses. Bennet above all favoured evacuation through the skin, not solely for Distillation but also for incipient Phthisis . It is accepted that, for internal gangrene, experienced physicians prescribe massage [frictions] & diaphoretic medicines, so that putrid matter in the blood may be drawn to the skin; and indeed reason and experience dictate that, where circulation has been increased through cutaneous vessels, there must be a revulsion from the praecordia; indeed the praecordia, already impeded, needs to make greater effort. If one adds what has been said already about normal perspirable matter, and that it will itself alone exceed in quantity all other evacuations produced at the same time, it will be agreed that it is of the utmost importance to promote perspiration through the skin: to this end a light diet helps and in a phrase, the use of the six nonnatural things,[12] which specifically promote perspiration, as Sanctorius observed. First and foremost, cold is to be avoided lest it constrict the skin pores. For Hippocrates said (recommending exercise as a cure) that great care must be taken that the patient should not become chilled, keeping near a fire in winter. He was to wear thicker clothing and sleep well covered with blankets, receiving massage in a warm room. Here too all forms of exercise and equitation greatly increase sweating, not only of benefit in lung conditions, but in many others to be mentioned later.

Almost all acridities may be evacuated by sweating; even those so fixed and solid that they cannot be expelled in the form of breath; besides, naturally acrid substances are always eliminated by the skin through sweating; if therefore the sweat of a completely healthy man, oozing drop by drop through the skin, is tasted, it will seem to be strongly tainted with acridity. Sweating may be encouraged by anything which increases circulation, by diminishing resistance in the skin vessels or by altering the flow of blood in them, especially if at the same time fluids are at hand capable of filtering through the cutaneous vessels. The first method scarcely applies, since bloodflow increases almost equally in the interior of the body as in the skin. Resistance in the skin may be diminished where vessels are locally relaxed and open. In this respect nothing deserves more recommendation than a steam bath.

Flow of blood through the skin is governed by external heat, which can be applied by degrees with a dry stove; my own preference is the cistella sudatoria, the head remaining free, allowing warm but unpolluted air to be drawn in to the lungs, which also derive benefit; I am sure also, for providing heat, that the steam bath is particularly beneficial. Massage may be added to those agents increasing blood flow through the skin. Thin aromatic drinks: as infus. & decoct. quinque rad. aperient. &c,[13] may be warmed and sipped; the skin vessels relax internally, being gently stimulated, restoring their contents; hot water always acts in this way, particularly if a weak stimulant is added, either washing out acrimony, or if of a contrary nature to the acrimony, overcoming it, and replenishing the thin humour lost in sweat. Sweating must be induced with care. Balnea humida, which relax the skin vessels, are of use where skin is tight and body type is more tense; dry heat indeed is better for those more relaxed and these too benefit by Massage. Sweating induced in the morning, when perspiration is greatest, or in the evening, to the point of dampness as with light dew, in accordance with the invalid's strength and repeated often, is much to be recommended.

The skin is thoroughly cleansed by Sweating, ensuring perspiration is not hindered later by blockage of cutaneous vessels with oily substances. A thin humour should be at hand to replace the diffused liquid, lest the blood becomes excessively viscous. The skin may be affected by itching spots when acrid sweats break out, even so disease may be relieved by this method which ought to be used more often.

Acrimony of the blood may be subdued by testing its nature with remedies opposed to it; these are commonly known as specifics, and produce an easier and quicker cure. Natural acrimonies must be grouped together with their opposing remedies, as indicated by faults in the humours; indeed there are general remedies which weaken almost every kind of acrimony, in particular those which dilute and others which cause viscosity; the only true diluent is water, the allimportant solvent in saline, by this the most venomous poison can be harmlessly drunk after dilution; beyond doubt every kind of acrimony miscible with water may with this be washed out from the blood; yet whatever causes pain may so weaken the body that it can scarcely endure it. If the acrimony is mixed intimately with oily humours, it is flushed out only with difficulty by aqua simplici. Here various saponaceous agents are added, varying with the natures of the acrimonies present; the humours then, after removal of acridities, should be restored to that delicate state where, miscible with water, they can flow through small vessels acting as organs of excretion. Agents causing viscosity either blunt sharp spicules or cover them with a sheath; these include viscosa, balsamica, emollientia, oleosa, blanda, decocta & condita limacum; all make the acrimony sticky and weak, enabling nature to overcome it; besides this it provides a remarkable source of nourishment; amongst all these gifts mucilaginibus gum. arabic. & tragacanth. are in many ways to be preferred. Most desirable also are soups and decoctions of river crabs for bland and soothing nourishment; other remedies are wellknown; examples are the following: of the emollientia & mucosa the best are consolida, althaea, cum toto, sem. lini, hordeum;[14] with regard to healing herbs glycyrrhiza should be mentioned, but balsamicum too is very suitable. Among bland oils are those from sweet almonds (recently expressed), and from spermaceti, pistachios and pine kernels.

From these and similar preparations in the shops one may collect all kinds of decocta, emulsiones, linctus, & formulae. There is however one drawback, these remedies, equally with diluents, can only be used if prescribed in large quantities, which certainly weakens the body intensely, causing lax vessels, from which harm may arise later; but they may be taken in these larger quantities without harm if at the same time stimulants & astringents are prudently introduced. By stimulant I mean that which increases the circulation of the blood; this may be by physical movement, exercise &c, substances swallowed, either foods or medicines, by applications, such as massage or baths; anything that can produce this effect. Astringents are known by their taste; one can tell both stimulants and astringents by their effect. None seems to strengthen the vessels as much as steel.

It is possible to combine all in one formula; for example that prescribed by Bennet for Haemoptysis arising from inborn acrimony of the blood; all, with few exceptions used for other purposes, comprise astringents, gentle stimulants, & emollients, varied as the occasion demands.

The simpler method of Hippocrates & Sydenham, already mentioned, is much favoured: raw cow's milk, mixed with a third part of honey and water, to be drunk over a period of forty five days, mixed with origano (in a communal draught if one wishes). Also wine should be considered, harsh and black, as old and pleasant as possible, but in moderation: they also recommended exercise. Truthfully, to profit by all this these remedies must be used long and assiduously, following the precepts of Hippocrates.

As far as the lungs are concerned, if the distillation was due to laxity or weakness, they may be strengthened locally by suffumigra gummi;[15] this is heated over a glowing coal and the fumes inhaled with the aid of an upturned funnel, for preference with the instrument designed for this by Bennet; eminently suitable for fumigation in this way are mastich., oliban., styrax calamit., sarcocolla & succinum[15]; the effect of these is to dilate the openings of the vessels through which very thick humours trickle into narrowed bronchi and strengthen the whole structure of the bronchi and vesiculae. The effect of such suffumigation may daily be tested for arresting Coryza, yet this cure is better preceded by frequent evacuations.

It may be that the lungs are badly strained by coughing, resulting in many severe ills; many large convulsions and constrictions may occur, forcing humours into alien vessels, which at any time may break asunder; free and even circulation through the lungs is impeded and sleeplessness and other symptoms may arise; for which reason I believe that a cough, if severe, must be quietened by some means before elimination. Emollientia & balsamica soothe cough to some extent but the virtues of opium provide the sacred anchor.

Certain other matters should be mentioned. If excessive Fever arises, or Plethora is present, bleeding is indicated, as the occasion demands. This way Haemoptysis may be prevented, medication made more effective, and circulation of humours freed; so acrimony flows with greater ease or is expelled. If nature deposits diseased material anywhere one must avoid everything that disturbs it and lead it off by suitable channels. Walking is to be encouraged, even more than horseriding in fact, and Willis was certainly right to recommend travel in warmer climates. Again a communal medicinal drink of water and milk to which may be added honey and a pinch of cinnamon, mace, lemon peel, or else aromatic hyssop may be used; or red wine, in moderation, if there is no fear of fever. Instead of this communal cup, Bennet suggested medicinal beer, also to be recommended for its total nourishment with which he aptly and clearly treated this condition. He imposed strict diet for Haemoptysis from acrimony of the blood. Sleep needs great encouragement, for nothing favours acrid humours so much as restlessness. All fatty, hot and acrid foods are to be avoided, as Hippocrates dictated, echoed by Bennet. Sydenham, on the other hand, forbade spirituous liquors and meat, especially where there is a tendency to Fever.

I have spoken at length about acrid Distillation because a slight increase in the disease is full of danger; herein are the true essentials for curing any kind of Haemoptysis and Phthisis.

Concerning cogestion due to pituitous, cold and viscous phlegm

Under this heading I beg to include all obstructions of the lungs produced by cold pituitous, or crude and glutinous matter, with no inflammation, together with its ejection by cough.

It is known that in a mild climate pituitous matter is cold, with a limpid colour; it goes with heaviness and torpor of body, apathy, prolonged sleep and a tendency to doze. This follows a crude diet of glutinous foods, especially in unhealthy amounts, the body becoming accustomed to inactivity; the stomach containing much crude matter, pale and unformed, causes a swollen abdomen: one may suspect crude chyle is beginning to cause obstruction in the lung by very troublesome breathlessness and cough when chyle is mixing with the blood: obstruction from any viscous or cold humour results in uncomfortable heaviness of the chest, a feeling as if a stone is lying on it; also pain in the back and irksome cough, especially in the aged; sputa are thick and firm, of varying colour, whitish, clear, bluish, blackish, rusty, now in round discs, now irregular. Often great effort produces no expectoration despite irritation and strain; this is easier after a rich meal, more difficult in humid weather; likewise invalids are prone to breathlessness on exercise or bodily movement; a fit of coughing may at any time induce dread of suffocation, always worse after cold or viscous foods; this condition improves in summer, but gets worse when it is cold or humid; strong indications of this disease in which Bennet described the breathing as truly resembling a pendulum clock, repeatedly swinging to and fro.

Here the immediate cause seems to be raw and sticky humour, filling pulmonary vessels and obstructing flow, thence at any time displaced into the bronchial cavity, the bounty of nature. Is it actually compacted at this point while being forced in to the bronchi? Or is it actually stagnating there, acquiring the thick consistency of sputum? One cannot be certain. The very narrow vessels and the need for pulmonary and bronchial passages to allow free flow, supports the latter view; in fact experiments show that even very thick material is probably expelled through these passages.

So dense inflammatory matter occupying lungs or settling in some other part of the chest is removed, with complete eradication of the disease; without this process Hippocrates (who so roundly condemned dry Peripneumonia and Pleurisies) believed a proper cure to be almost impossible; purulent abscesses of the chest are also drained in this way: on which Aretaeus, taught by Hippocrates, writes as follows: 'after this has occurred (concerning lung abscess), there is no need for the strain and effort of evacuation as required in solid parts of the body': pus is expelled readily, distension occurring more easily in these very fine vessels than in the general structure of the body; for the lung is thin, full of cavities like a sponge; not injured by the humour, it moves it constantly into passages of increasing width, finally reaching the trachea; the same applies to Asthmas arising from glutinous material, ejection of much purulent and moist sputum being a healthy sign; from this disease it is clear how material, unable to flow through pulmonary vessels, is forced down into the bronchi.

Because of this it is believed that the lungs are chiefly freed by thick sputa allowing restoration of the normal kind of material present in the lung.

This is the essence of this disease, origins are more remote; that which generates viscous humour and that which predisposes the lungs to this condition. The first group stems from bad coction in the first passages associated with dull or glutinous diet; or lack of the essential attrition of heart and arteries, the causes being legion; excessive withdrawal of the more subtle humours of the lung, indeed anything preventing free transit induces disease more quickly in that part; such, for example, as narrowness of vessels in lung malformation; destruction of tissue by progressive disease; or narrowing of vessels by excessive rigidity occuring in old age.

On the other hand, the opposite faults of laxity and weakness produce the same effect; here vessels are very prone to yield to the humours and dilate, then those first receiving blood from larger vessels compress those in the vicinity, reducing the numbers available; through the dilated openings of the side vessels humours pass to unfavourable ones and obstruct them; and even those unaffected in this way lack the power of their own elasticity, so necessary for expelling the humours they contain; hence obstructions of all kinds arise, so it is clear why the old, and the youthful but inactive (especially females), who eat crude viscous food, are prone to this disease rather than Tabes and Haemoptysis .

There is a possible objection to this opinion, for Hippocrates attributes this disease to 'απο τυλαιπωριης',[16] which all interpreters have rendered as 'labour'; if the true nature of the disease is carefully considered, that it is very slow, remitting in summer, that cough disturbs chiefly the aged, that complexion is fresh, and breathlessness may result, so it seems that 'misery' is really a better word, implying an inherent sadness of heart; thus circulation of the humours becomes more languid and a defect occurs in the essential attrition of heart and vessels. On the other hand there are those illnesses which do arise from toil, or physical effort; all varieties, both inflammatory and 'acute', for which the main remedy is rest, truly in our view to be described as labour. I do not believe that labour is what is intended here, unless this implies sickness or some ill effect; in that sense indeed Hippocrates very often used the word 'πόνος'.[16]

Prognosis here was set down by Hippocrates, who told us that a slow, burdensome condition, lasting as much as three years, was very likely to be fatal; for a viscous humour, forced into the vessels, produces tubercles in the lungs, crude and frigid, stagnating slowly and becoming acrid; surrounding vessels are eroded, producing an abscess or concealed ulcer. This indeed is how ulcers are formed, rarely single but very commonly multiple. Also there is dread of suffocation by humour obstructing the vessels and impeding crossflow of humours through the lungs; this, in the opinion of Aretaeus, occurs from slow Congestion, but often from fever or violent cough. Furthermore, even with strong circulation, pulmonary vessels may be narrow, weak and delicate; excessively crude and glutinous chyle, may block capillary vessels: this causes Dyspnoea and rapid onset of Haemoptysis from a ruptured vessel.

Cure aims at dissolving, diluting and attenuating excessively viscous and obstructive humours; and by drawing stagnant humours into the circulation, or removing them, then dealing with the causes of the disease as far as one can.

Therefore, if agreed that the first passages are flooded with viscous fluid, a common event where disease arises from bad coction, they will have first priority in treatment, ensuring that disease is not constantly fuelled, and the way is free for medication and chyle; so the first passages, stimulated and restored, ensure complete coction; for this, matter must first be liquefied, then evacuated. First of all remedies used are saponacea,[17] chosen for their ability to stimulate the stomach and flaccid, inert intestines; also supplying a deficiency of bile, invariably lacking; they are opposed to the essence of the disease, which indeed tends to acidity; soaps act because they are made of alkaline salts and oil; of these there is none better than sapone veneta; almost as good are gummi saponacea, amarescentia & aromatica; examples of these are asafoetida, ammoniacum, sagapenum, galbanum opopanax, bdellium, myrrha, and others with this inherent quality: juices also, such as bitter herbs beginning to ferment, are particularly suitable: excellent remedies are thickened animal bile & oxymel scilliticum. Much inertia of stomach and intestines needs greater stimulation, here one may add sales alkalini fortes, bulbi recent. ari, flores benzoin; and from these one may derive various formulae; many are exhibited in solid form, but liquids may be more convenient.

These and similar agents render matter more fluid and easily expelled by natural means; but in an accumulation in the stomach an evacuation is possible with emetics such as vinum benedictum cum oxymelle scillitico; if lower down purgatives are preferred, as long as the intestines have not been weakened nor adversely affected by disease; suitable agents are aloe, preparations of which include elix. propriet. pilul. coch., & hiera picra; also, theriac, diatesseron of Mesue, rheum & fructus myrobalan,[18] which strengthen the intestines; the dose such that the bowel is moved gently three or four times each day: purgatives are less suitable for the elderly.

When this has been done one must try to banish all this viscosity from the blood vessels; the action of remedies being suggested is by no means directed at the first passages alone, though that aim suffices; other helpful remedies may be introduced as reinforcements and their use continued; and, as has been said, one may drink liquid after the aperient; it is possible to use extracts from many plants, cichoraceis, rad. aperient. and lignis sasafr., trium santalor;[19] also juice may be expressed from alkalescent herbs, antiscorbutics, and those for cleansing and healing, providing infusions and decoctions that meet immediate needs; it may be desirable to add sal. polycrest. & honey: also medicinal wines with fixed alkaline vegetable salts in solution, and balsamorum pectoralium; maximum use of blistering agents is wise, such as cantharides; decoctum ligni guaici simplex, suitably applied, is totally reliable.

Exercise enhances treatment, at first as much as is easily borne, increasing gradually to the desired level; regular physical movement is of great importance, especially with regard to the chest, and here equitation is supreme; here too massage is recommended, with similar precautions; personally I consider it most important that the patient should be exposed to a dry stove, after decoctions of recommended ligni, as much as he can absorb; he should be warmed by slow degrees until it is seen that a slight fever occurs and some sweating, if considered desirable; the invalid's strength and other signs will indicate the level of heat and its duration; then he may be rubbed down well after sweating. If there has been some previous neglect, I might order decocto guiaci every fourth day, with the dry stove at intervals; the object being to cause a barely perceptible fever, reduced when deemed sufficient; in this way the whole paroxysm may be completed in about six hours, the patient's strength being sustained with a nourishing diet.

Finally, to complete this matter, if the patient's body is lax and Leucophlegmatic, only debilated with no obstruction, the best remedy is pilul. gummos: ferrum.

Nature, as we see, is slow to dissolve thick humour blocking vessels, promoting greater circulation or, the same thing, fever; this is also induced by stimulants, exercise and massage. A currently used method of sweating, much commended, follows nature, emulating as far as art can the paroxysms of quartan fever; this, as is known to physicians, relieves many chronic diseases and overcomes visceral obstructions. Further, by the same method, slightly varied, all humours may be dissolved and expelled through the skin pores; also, very delicate vessels, such as occur in marrow and at the very edge of the circulation, may be flushed and purged; as examples of this, Lues venerea, which feeds off the bones, and Spina ventosa, are both cured by this method; albeit if any doubt exists about the ability of this treatment to cure this disease, one may look to Bennet; he confirmed this method in his own practice, introducing the use of mercurial medicines.

Concerning the order and method of using these remedies, it is not possible to be specific, until the condition of the patient has been agreed; in general one can say that if there is lax bodily makeup, verging on Leucophlegmasia, the use of liquids should be more sparing and sweating by dry heat is required more often; here too muscular exercise is very suitable. The aged should be given exercises which cause least loss of breath, requiring less effort. Circulation is gradually to be stimulated with utmost discretion; lest material, at present unable to pass through is forced more firmly into the vessels, with new obstructions in the lungs and so suffocation; indeed healing must proceed gently and smoothly, for the disease requires slow and lengthy treatment.

Diet, which should be considered first, is of utmost importance; who benefits by all this treatment if crude chyle causes continual new obstructions? Food should be easily digested, nutritious, passing easily through the vessels and opposed to the morbid diathesis; firstly, the most suitable types of food are meat soups with biscuit, with uncooked roots and aromatic herbs to act as aperients; but if the patient is of a leucophlegmatic type a drier diet is preferable, mainly biscuit with wellcooked tender meats, taken with spiced wine. Fasting from time to time is desirable, either by having smaller meals or omitting them altogether. As a drink, wellfermented beer from bitter hops, and noble white wine of the kind that comes from the Canary islands; or, if fibres are lax, red or black wines, rough or wellbred, are suitable. All farinaceous, and raw foods from vegetables that have not been well softened, or are rough and unripe, are to be avoided, likewise glutinous and fatty food, selected from animal parts. Patients should take less sleep and avoid exposing themselves to cold and damp.

Lastly, finally to dispose of this matter, if malformation of the lung or the rigidity of old age have disposed the body to this disease. nothing can be done; the illness can certainly be inhibited by diet, and the six nonnaturals, used as already stated. Excessive laxity of the vessels may be cured by strengthening medicines, preferably those which contain iron, but chiefly by exercise.

Disease, arising from obstructed vessels is not very different from that described; when Fever, bodily exertion, or some other cause provokes violent circulation of the humours, exhalant bronchial vessels, by stretching out the follicles placed there, are so dilated that they accept a humour thicker than normal; the humour being so viscous and the force propelling it so feeble that flow cannot occur, would seem to be the root of the disease.

Sydenham noticed that this illness arose after fevers and was particularly troublesome in the aged; here perhaps an added cause is the narrowing of the vessels or their openings into the bronchi or, even more, the follicles; this may happen during winter, when after violent exercise the body is exposed incautiously to much cold; the humour stagnates, blocked in these vessels and cavities; the more liquid part is reabsorbed (mainly by the follicles), and the rest compressed into pultaceous material, almost chalky in fact, which in some way restores the cavities of the follicles; perhaps the acridity and resulting weakness excite cough; if not successfully relieved through sputum, if it does not diminish, or is not absorbed by other vessels, a purulent abscess will then form.

If the smallest lung vessels become overfilled, without other great damage, one should prescribe medicines which dissolve congested material: for example, sapo venetus, decocta ex rad. & herbis aperientibus, cum sale polycrest; for nourishment meat broth, for drinking good quality wine & balsamicum ; these and physical exercise, happily complete the cure for very many people.

Concerning haemoptysis

Haemoptysis is the expulsion of blood from the lungs through the mouth; blood ejected upwards will be known to have come from the lungs if it occurs with a deep hawking or cough and the throwing up of frothy material or of a bright red or florid colour.

Blood from the lungs may come from two sources, from dilated peripheral vessels or those continually being broken down.

In Haemoptysis from the spreading out of the vessels or from anastomoses, a Greek term, blood is seldom ejected continually and in full flow; but sputa are often bloody or streaked with blood; blood may flow for a limited time, in which case no malaise, pain, or pressure on the chest are felt, or only very little; such sputa are produced by hawking for an hour or two after waking in early morning; sometimes with other symptoms erupting in the afternoon, or may accompany morning cough, as often with acrid distillation. Also blood formerly lost at intervals in other ways sometimes takes this path; thus menstrual blood is often lost through blood stained sputum, lasting three or four days and stopping without any remedy, until menstruation starts again.

This disease may be caused by laxity of vessels, remembering the force of the bloodflow (explaining the frequency of haemoptysis in men living in high mountains); more often it is attributable to a certain natural diathesis.

The integrity of vessels is damaged by erosion, laceration, or both. Erosion may occur from acrid humour destroying the vessels which contain it; also from acrid Catarrh, Ulceration of lung, or else from certain acrid poisons; here the bleeding is continuous, the amount related to the size of eroded vessels;

164

acrid Catarrh in its early stages can erode many minor vessels, the blood-stained sputa tasting salty.

Damage to vessels may occur at any time without warning, when coughing or during great exertion: perhaps from some other cause, approaching more stealthily, impeding free flow of blood through the lungs: Haemoptysis may occur with other barely perceptible signs, slight discomfort, moderate warmth, a flushed face, and some breathing difficulties, as if the chest is constricted. Eventually blood appears, as described, with cough and rattling of the lung; often it flows in little waves, so that as Aretaeus said, it seems rather to be vomited than expectorated; blood erupting in bronchi may form membranous clots, often regarded by Physicians as membranes investing the bronchi and the very vessels of the lung; Ruysch however deduced that these came from agitated blood, having noted the same appearance in blood formed in the uterus. It is certain sometimes that the actual blood vessels are expectorated, following a previous erosion. of which Tulp gives one or two examples; but acrid Catarrh always precedes it. The pulse in Haemoptysis is soft, weak, and wavering, accompanied by breathlessness and if a salty taste in the mouth precedes it it is a sign that a saline acrimony has reached the lungs.

The less common causes of Haemoptysis can be reduced to three heads; weakness and frailty of pulmonary vessels, increased force of blood in the vessels, and acrimony of the blood.

(1) The pulmonary vessels cannot be other than weak and frail where all vessels are very close together; this may be suspected by slenderness of body, pellucid skin, high colour and a pleasant flush. Here at any time a source of trouble may be set up in the lungs, or it may always have been there, indicating a hereditary taint. The vessels finally become enfeebled by progressive disease, usually acrid Catarrh.

(2) The thrust of the blood on the pulmonary vessels is increased by Plethora, which occurs most often when the body reaches its physical peak; from this comes the Hippocratic observation: 'In young people Haemoptysis occurs mainly from the eighteenth year to the thirty sixth'; an age when he particularly expected all critical haemorrhages. This happens if the blood circulation is greatly increased, particularly where blood has reached its final destination in the lungs; for example, a sudden coldness constricting the outer surface of the body, from tight clothing or immersion in water; another cause might be some great strain, or repeated muscular effort, or from jumping, from high altitudes, by the lifting of heavy weights or certain other kinds of violent exercise &c.

Further causes might be a condition of pulmonary vessels, where flow of blood is impeded; likewise rigidity of vessels by disease or by nature, from drinking quantities of cold water, from strong contraction of the muscles of expiration, perhaps voluntarily, as with the effort of long straining at stool;

from singing and shouting, the muscular spasms of vomiting, laughing &c; spasm of the intercostal muscles, as when cold, acrid, or astringent air is breathed in; pulmonary vessels are damaged not only by disease and viscous humour, especially chyle, obstructing many delicate vessels, but by external compression of the chest; natural narrowing of pulmonary vessels goes with a badly shaped chest and that hinders free expansion of the lungs; finally from thick matter blocking and distending pulmonary vesicles and perhaps the bronchi.

These are the signs that free circulation through the lungs is impeded: difficult, gasping respiration, an oppressive feeling in the chest, a hot flushed appearance, visible pulsation in the carotid artery and often slight vertigo; these are greatly aggravated by bodily movement and increased circulation; similarly with narrowing of the pulmonary vessels, a common reason for transflow being blocked; the situation becomes more serious four to six hours after food, particularly if raw, or where large amounts have been eaten, together with mild fever and a light dry cough.

(3) Acrimony of the humours may be closely related to the last group, because it is believed that acrimony arises from spicules, humours becoming acrid when round particles become pointed; assuming this, it may be shown that such a moving body may penetrate another, especially if travelling deeply: moreover the round particles in humours easily slip by the walls of the vessels, whereas the angular must fix in them, being forced in more deeply by continual propulsion to the heart: this acrimony may be known for its bloodred colour, shining most beautifully through the vessels; indeed from its thin, dilute composition any circulating blood is hardly able to form clots and gives off an odour of ammonia. The causes thus range from diathesis to acrid catarrh and all else already stated. For this reason Haemoptysis often follows putrid scurvy, putrid fevers, particularly smallpox and plague.

Finally, there may be a break in continuity of vessels by a wound of the thorax, perhaps by a rigid, sharp object penetrating the bronchi, or a hard, spiky calculus forming there.

Where several factors act together, the more quickly Haemoptysis occurs; my sedulous enquiries into these matters have been intended to identify possible predisposing causes, or at least to give awareness of warning signs.

Authors have made great distinctions between disease from blood flowing from bronchial vessels and that from pulmonary vessels; the chief difference lies in the ability of both kinds of vessel to withstand attack; but small branches make anastomoses everywhere, as shown by the skill of Ruysch, who injected the pulmonary vessels, distending them; it is possible to pass from the right side of the heart through bronchial vessels into the bronchial cavity. If blood is ejected by light hawking, in small quantities, not as yet florid and without any discomfort in the chest, it is assumed to have trickled from the lining of the windpipe: if sputa containing bloody mucus are produced through coughing it is from the membrane lining the bronchus.

Where there is deep, irritating cough, however, pure blood, florid and copious is expectorated at brief intervals; coughing may have been preceded by a feeling of suffocation, and succeeded by a sense of greater freedom by the eruption from these same vessels.

Haemoptysis from injury to the windpipe is slight; a lesion of vessels of the bronchial membrane is worse; even worse where it has come from a pulmonary vessel: but if it arises from simple dilatation of vessels with no Cacochymia there is often no great harm, though always a danger of more disruption.

Bloody, salty sputum from acrid Distillation may be expectorated some-times for years, but it is very dangerous unless very careful cure is instituted. Heavy loss of blood, perhaps daily, may lead to pituitous Cacochymia, creating a putrescent ulcer; blood insinuating itself between the membranes of the lung may lead to a false aneurism.

Phthisis, almost always due to erosion, follows preexisting disease, mainly malformation of the lungs and hereditary taint; attacking at a certain age, it is cured with difficulty, but Haemoptysis is a cause for concern; when occurring from breakage of a major vessel it results in sudden suffocation, or brings syncope from loss of blood, and then death. In putrid fevers it is always lethal. Finally, Haemoptysis is always to be feared lest it results in the forma-tion of a lung ulcer.

The disease is certainly of the utmost danger, from which there are few survivors. On the other hand, a well-built man if previously in perfect health, especially if he is square-chested, well-rounded and breathes freely, deeply and slowly, may expect nothing too serious from this malady; with a good remedy he may escape: free breathing, sedation of cough, and the restoration of strength after Haemoptysis increase hope. If slimy sputum, blue and light, continues after the bloodstaining, it shows that the disease may recur in the future in young, warmblooded people.

Haemoptysis may be cured by dilatation of vessels; this averts or quietens bloodflow in the lungs, subdues acrimony of the blood and strengthens pulmonary vessels. Suitable remedies are those customarily used for cure of acrid Catarrh and I therefore omit them; I add only that blood is to be let more boldly, and repeatedly; and stimulants of the circulation must used very cautiously. If blood, normally lost through other channels, reaches the lungs, those channels must be reopened; delay may cause immediate plethora, so blood must be removed by venesection at a convenient site: plethora is always to be avoided. If ever it accompanies acrid Catarrh it may be avoided by sweating in the cistella. The pulmonary vessels should never be strength-ened by deep breathing, unless fourteen days has passed since the Haemoptysis has settled.

With more copious Haemoptysis or circulation much increased there is a case for letting blood very freely; depending on the patient's temperature and strength, up to four times a day or more if Haemoptysis still continues after an interval; if the disease has almost settled, blood must be extracted repeatedly over a long period but in gradually smaller amounts, and at longer intervals, or whenever plethora and vigour return; this may weaken the patient, so one should beware of Cacochymia from lack of blood.

If there is anxiety about excessive loss of blood, ligatures may be applied to the limbs, afterwards to be gradually loosened. Clothing which is too tight should be removed at once and for a time the invalid confined to bed, or else abstain as much as possible from muscular movement and emotional excitement, speaking little, and with a quiet voice; he should not breathe deeply: cough certainly should be sedated with syr. diacodii. The surface of the body should be relaxed with a steam bath, to the extremities at least, and by relaxing fomentations; gentle heat does no harm, but cold must be kept out by thick blankets, taking very great care, since as much harm is to be feared from their pressure as from the cold; in this regard it is possible for pressure on the body to be prevented by blanket supports: the air should be temperate and humid; the bowel should be kept loose, if it becomes costive a bland enema may be given so that strains on the abdomen are prevented.

All food should be cold, easily digested, passing easily through all vessels, bland and nourishing: there is nothing better than milk and water, but if natural vigour is strong, then whey; one may order emulsions from bland cereals and from oily flour products, panatellae, particularly made from biscuit; juice, cream, ptisane, rice, barley, millet and oats; rice is preferable because it is savoury, easily digestible without salt or condiment. Fruits in season, properly ripe, cooked to relieve flatulence, are to be encouraged; if the body is weak, diluted meat broth may be allowed, to which has been added a little orange juice in place of salt; small meals taken in between may be of benefit as long they are not acidforming. All these things should be in small quantities and continually varied, of foremost importance in allowing easy flow through pulmonary vessels. When vessels are hard and thickened with scar tissue they must be gradually and slowly relaxed by this method of healing, guarding against Cacochymia and loss of blood; at all times the patient must abstain from acrid, spirituous and stimulating substances, and similarly from everything of a viscous or obstructive nature; from any one of these Haemoptysis may return. Plethora is to be guarded against above all. So, unless the Haemoptysis is congenital or incurable, the disease itself gives the first warning.

One may wonder that many remedies of great repute have been omitted, such as styptics or the specifics I have mentioned. Styptics I have discovered are caustic and either clot the blood or thicken it or contract the vessels; but topical application of these may be admissible to some extent; for this they must be inhaled through the mouth to the lungs or introduced into the body and thus able to exert an even effect on venous vessels in the lungs; no more needs to be said on this. Specifics indeed deserve to be considered, lapis haematit., sanguis draconis, terra pingues & adstringentes, or bolus armena, terra lemnia, sigillatae &c;[20] the first of these deserves commendation but on the whole I judge it to be harmful unless the main cause of the disease is excessive laxity of the vessels; though the purest mineral iron, use in daily practice is a mistake; the iron of the blood may increase the force of the circulation, therefore it is certainly opposed to all those things that we depend on, such as S.M.,[21] watery diet &c. The others do not seem to be detrimental but there is no great expectation of good from that direction; they may be used after deliberation, so that thereafter no physician may be blamed by jealous or ignorant people alleging that the best remedy has been omitted or ignored.

Thickening of the fluids has indeed been mentioned, being already viscous, and obstructing the capillary vessels of the lung. These vessels being disrupted, no glutinous or meaty food may be given. If one requires a specific remedy, this may be found in the opiates; but a diligent search for them is often vain; for, truth to tell, syr. de meconio is not very potent, other than in the sedation of cough; but in the opinion of Sydenham, even in bleeding from the nose, V.S [venesection][22] needing ligatures and many other situations it has been found wanting; he placed his greatest hope in paregoric after venesection, for blood in the urine, or the bloody sputum of smallpox, taken once nightly; and also in those haemorrhages where the blood may be staunched at the wound, unless there is some minor obstacle, which opium relieves by free circulation of the humours; or perhaps there may be some other reason for its good effect on which I will not venture an opinion.

Concerning pulmonary phthisis

I now turn to the subject of Phthisis; a sequel to ulcer of the lung, hence the term pulmonary. It is known that the establishment in the lung of this disease develops gradually, along with vague anxiety and slowly increasing breathlessness; if there is a concealed abscess there will be dry cough (sputa at this stage are not purulent, but of normal appearance); there is also a sense of weight on the chest, flushing of cheeks, and low hectic fever occurring four to six hours after food; at this stage the most serious of the various symptoms. Thirst is greater than normal, there is weight loss and weakness; all early signs of disease, with daily deterioration. Pus stagnates in the lung, becoming more acrid, eroding neighbouring vessels and slowly destroying its substance ; the abscess grows, firing the tinder which damages all humours, leading to Atrophy and death: in this way a great part of the lung is destroyed or else the abscess breaks into the air passages and the patient dies, suffocated by corrupt matter. In other cases pus is ejected by coughing, its quantity and nature indicating the size and type of abscess, or it may collect in the thoracic cavity, resulting in an Empyema. One must admit, however, that though pus is made in the lungs, this may not seem to be the case when a man is suffocating from a throat infection.

If there is an open ulcer, either from a ruptured abscess, an erosion, or another cause, there may be many signs added to those of hidden abscess; morning and afternoon cough, with a variety of sputa, as so often stated, (this is the most important sign, save where sputa are purulent after Haemoptysis, from blood stagnating in the lung with no ulcer); such sputa may be light, even, white, dried up, or sweetish - all more favourable; or else bilious, compact, round, uneven, fatty, greyish, rusty, thin, bloody, less good: the worst indeed are stringy, dirty, foetid, claylike, and certain more liquid kinds, the heaviest of all, which sink in salt water. As with sputum, blood may at any time be eroded from the substance of the lungs and expelled.

Apart from sputa, the signs of Phthisis (many, developing all the time) are these: foetid breath, pain in the chest, sore nipples exacerbated by coughing, increasing difficulty in breathing; hectic fever, noticeably worse at night and fading by first light, weak, slow pulse and warmth in the upper parts from acridity, lips and face becoming flushed; great thirst and sweating at night; extreme anxiety coincides with the onset of fever: a host of misfortunes follow, total wasting away of the body, flesh vanishing and bony articulations and processes protruding everywhere; the nails are incurved and the facies described by Hippocrates is plain to see (Aretaeus thus vividly described the image of death); feet swell, and sometimes hands, there is great weakness and red pustules and hoarse voice may be present.

Finally there is an exudation of fluid from the capillaries, itching over the whole body, and watery blisters; these are full of thin, acrid humours; they can no longer be kept apart from vessels and often break through into the intestine; this causes yellow Diarrhoea, foetid, purulent, more liquid as sputum diminishes; almost always this opens the doorway to the house of death.

Knowledge passed down makes understanding easy; how Atrophy occurs from lung ulcer, open or concealed: for wherever lung function is stricken, crude matters may not be digested and from that glowing tinder humours draw taint to themselves; the first effect of this is starvation of humours, the body being drained by the copious sputum.

The symptoms of Phthisis are easily explained: hectic fever arises at a fixed time after meals, when chyle enters the blood, humours increasing in quantity and crude ones accumulating in the lungs; of these a part is already damaged, but in the greater part function has not been disturbed; humours pass through with difficulty, thick ones being retained, especially in those vessels prone to ulceration; hence obstruction and creation of moderate inflammation; cough and dyspnoea increase, inducing anxiety: such fever lasts until inflammation is resolved and the flow of obstructing materials restored, by drainage through the ulcer (hence sputa concocted by morning fever are copious), or until the expulsion of most other humours; when thin these disperse easily through skin pores; since desirable lung function requires thrust and flexibility, they may now no longer have the required strength and tenacity, being light and moist; besides, the humours flooding out are largely destroyed by purulent material mixed with them; they are forced with difficulty along proper channels, spreading laterally and causing night sweats; in due course watery Diarrhoea occurs, since the intestine drains away almost everything. Warmth of the upper parts and flushing of the face occurs because free descent of blood through the jugular veins is impeded; thirst is due to obstruction of the lung and acrimony of the humours; cough is caused by any source of bronchial irritation, such symptoms arise so easily.

Phthisis after hereditary Haemoptysis is the worst kind of all, healing is very difficult; the same applies to Empyema of the chest. Sputa, muddy, heavy &c, occur with all the signs of chronic Phthisis; other sputa may be white, sweet, like egg albumen becoming firm when heated; these are the very worst, especially following acrid Catarrh, with debility and general decay. If hectic fevers, fluctuating unevenly throughout the day, should plague the patient, the illness is surely lethal. Where pleurae are adherent to lung, death from Phthisis is certain. Death follows speedily the outpouring of capillary fluid as liquid diarrhoea. Swelling of the feet and hands and coldness of the extremities are all bad signs. Patients with phthisis who expectorate bland, ripe sputa, and also the elderly, withstand the disease better and survive longer; in those who excrete bilestained matter and in the young, life is shorter; and those succumb very rapidly who produce saline matter or of bad smell or taste.

Finally it should be said that all pulmonary Phthisis is intensely dangerous on account of the nature of the parts affected and because an ulcer is only removed with difficulty. If acrid Catarrh is present cure is not possible; it must be eradicated beforehand and all humours sweetened. Neither wound nor ulcer heal unless healthy humours flow into them, and humours from damaged lungs do not recover easily. If sputa are white, ripe, even, light, sweet, and easily expectorated; if hectic fever is absent so the invalid has a good appetite and digestion; if there is no great thirst, excretion is healthy and the faeces firm and equal in quantity to the intake of food; besides that if the patient is not too thin, has a square and hairy chest, a small sternum, is robust and well covered with flesh, then these are all good signs; this was the opinion of Hippocrates, who stated: 'Whoever has all these will be most likely to survive; whoever indeed has none is close to death: for women to avoid Tabes it is necessary that menstruation should be splendid and faultless.'

Curing a concealed abscess, depends on the time required for it to mature and rupture. Infection of the blood by pus, and harm arising in the humours from defective action of the vessels, are danger signals. Pus must be removed from the ulcer and this reduced to scar tissue. Finally, nourishment is to be ordered that is concocted most easily, will flow through the lungs, and opposed to the nature of the disease.

The abscess must now be matured, as elsewhere in the body, by those substances which stimulate circulation, mainly balsamica, incidentia &

aromatica,[23] and, when circulation is strong enough, by emollients and milky food. The abscess wall may be soothed locally through the bronchus and relaxed by steam inhalation quite often during the day; if this does not produce great relaxation of the vessels, a small cough may be provoked with rupture into the bronchi, this should be attempted, with all due care, either by voluntary coughing or inhalation of steaming vinegar.

Travelling in a carriage over rough and uneven roads and equitation must be considered: but before this Hippocrates liked to see the patient's belly well-filled, but discretely, so the diaphragm is not pushed upwards, disturbing the bronchi which enclose the cavity.

Pus may be prevented from corrupting the blood by removal of acridity through absorbent veins, separating and thickening it and preserving the humours against decay. About the way acrid material is evacuated, all has been said; but preferred above all others is removal through the skin, unless at any time nature provides another way, such as through kidneys, bowel, or ulcers elsewhere: one can confirm this proper evacuation from the observations of Hippocrates; for instance at that time of year when perspiration is likely to be impeded, and all tends to decay quickly (one sees red and inflamed throats; or stinging, acrid diarrhoea with tenesmus, or thin acrid discharges, dry cough &c, confining one to the house for a time); then Consumption is rife and those inclined to it are quickly laid low; if it is not overcome quite soon all may be expected to die without delay. Inviscantia & diluentia are particularly to be selected from amongst remedies already mentioned.

Lastly, humours contrary to the decay arising from pus are the most suitable for use; acidforming substances, lightly acidulated salines and gently antiseptic balsamics, natural balsams, resins, or healing herbs, already mentioned, may be chosen; prescribed whenever necessary and in any convenient form.

Harm caused by other humours arising from lung damage or attrition is equally common in sufferers from Phthisis and is very destructive, as has been mentioned; it is to be prevented, as far as art can, by reinforcing the action of those lung vessels still free, and the whole body; by freeing obstructions of any sort; and prescribing what is needed for nourishment, soon to be mentioned. Muscular movement achieves this end above all else though it may sometimes be impossible because of the patient's debility; its place may be taken by massage & travel; the advent of equitation has proved particularly useful, providing a change from other exercise, which may be preferable; it aids free and full respiration, unblocking and restoring the lungs, especially with a strong adverse wind to increase the motion; it is best with an empty belly and a body replete with decoctis balsamicus or after final digestion is complete; certainly to be avoided immediately after food.

Regarding various forms of exercise, I wish to say that Sydenham attributed so many benefits to equitation that he bravely declared that Phthisis, even if longstanding, would surely be cured by it; just as intermittent fevers respond to Peruvian bark, or Syphilis to mercury; all examples of heroic efforts.

It is tedious indeed to repeat everything that has been said on this subject, while the pages written by every teacher of Medicine can be so readily turned; this may be overcome, by the method of writing B.L.[24] against quoted passages, making it possible to reread them easily.

If the ulcer is to become firm, regeneration of lost vessels is needed ; but this is only possible in the way that they were formed in the first place: there is clear evidence that nature achieves this when good pus is formed in an ulcer. There is a way of dealing with pus in the Surgeon's operating room; here vessels of all kinds leading to an ulcer are opened and transmit a proper and healthy humour (if so desired or the ulcer is crude, malignant. or contaminated); the thinner constituent is soaked up through absorbent vessels, the rest thickened, becoming pus; wherever there is much bland and balsamic matter (just as spreadout mucus exposed to the air may curl up and disintegrate) there will be new vessels beneath, which if cherished may regenerate completely. Thus it becomes clear why venereal, scorbutic, and scabious ulcers or those found in Cacochymia, can be cured only with difficulty until Euchymia is restored: in no other way can this survive the constant oozing of acrid humour in the ulcer, for which reason Bennet avowed that erosion of the lung from acrid Catarrh is incurable without complete sweetening of the blood. For good pus to form in the ulcer, Cacochymia, whenever present, must be cured; Catarrh dripping into the lungs must be gradually drawn away to other parts .

Besides this, the ulcer must be cleansed, and treated according to its particular nature. First this may be done by restoring permeability to the vessels leading to the ulcer, either by dissolving the viscosity blocking them, or opening up halfclosed canals, stimulated by vital energy; this, as stated, is provided by decocta balsamica, and vulneraria, in a suitable mixture for the patient, as much as needed each day; or by physical movement, and by being dispersed through exercise, especially equitation; some means of sweating is to be recommended if the disease is not too longstanding; and massage by any reasonable method, thus a reassembly of measures already used.

The nature of the ulcer latent in the lung is disclosed by sputa, the patient's temperature, and other indications, present and to come.

Sputa ejected in the morning (when they are most likely to shift) are very thin, spreading, inert and insipid; they are cold and humid, indicating a lax and contaminated ulcer: the most knowledgeable Surgeons cure these by suppurantia & detergentia; these comprise balsamics and calefacients, such as refined Venetian terebinth, bee venom, root of Florentine iris &c; also vegetable and fossil astringents and gentle corrosives; from these one may select any suitable for Ulcer of the lung; balsamic herbs, steeped in water, or balsam itself, may be applied; when heated, the steam, full of virtue, may safely be drawn into the lungs; at the same time if some constriction is desired then sussitus gummi aromaticorum may be used: it is indeed pointless to use common astringents for this purpose, for their properties do not vaporize, as anyone tasting water distilled from astringent herbs may verify. In this respect Bennet seems to have erred. He devised various formulae for this purpose, rejecting single items which may have an even stronger detergent effect than those already mentioned: among these he named barley, solution of oak gall, tormentil, Armenian bole; these are however of no benefit. His ideas are certainly not to be commended, for the particular virtues of balsamics & aromatics would be lost by heating. In his view the best detergent seems to be auripigmentum,[25] administered like a resin in the form of an inhalation; but this is considered to be very poisonous and hence is not used by the Author himself, who puts his trust in Diascorides, Pliny and many more, Greek or Arab, all Princes in the medical arts. They rarely commended auripigmentum, instead sandarachen Graecorum[25] is preferably applied to sordid lung ulcers. Perhaps it may in due course be made harmless through experience, adapting its preparation and method of use, perhaps finally to be used under the joint name auripigmenti sandarache.

Scanty sputa, bloodstained and acrid, with a sense of discomfort, of heat, throbbing in the chest and cough are constant companions, especially if above average fever is present, a preexisting cause having caused inflammation; other sputa, laudable and welcome, show the ulcer to be inflamed, and there is free perspiration.

One cures inflammation of this sort by removal of each and every cause; by drinking either diluents, antiphlogistics, or emollients; it does not hurt in general to use purgans antiphlogisticum if its use is indicated; otherwise the Ulcer may be relaxed by steam or hot milk. Sputa are usually produced from the drying out of the ulcer or much constriction of vessels; they are cured by watery and emollient draughts. If great quantities of acrid sputa are formed, with signs of acrid Catarrh, suitable action should be taken.

Sometimes viscous sputa, and those which are tenacious, thick, whitish, bluish, grey, rusty, and a mixture of the cold and the pituitous, are only seldom expectorated and then with great effort; the cough may be almost suffocating and often stertorous, usually after cold, glutinous foods, indicating excessive slowness of the humours to dissolve and a need for circulation to be increased. Assistance with this has been mentioned in the case of pituitous and viscous Congestion; balsamica & stimulantia must also be used locally. Sputa that are excessively thick and viscous may have an opposite cause, certainly from overheating; all such are chiefly bilious, easily distinguished by the patient's temperature. Useful here are diluentia saponacea non stimulantia; the latter for example might be decoct. hordei cum oxymelle, or rob. sambuci: it should be noted in passing that almost all Phthisical people expectorate thick sputa after eating viscous food.

If the Ulcer is really sordid and putrid, the sputa will be of the same nature,

174

unequal, bloodstained, mottled and foetid, together with offensive breath. Any cacochymia must be hunted down and cured. Detergents are to be used to the full, both internally and externally, according to the type of Ulcer: if sputa are putrid even stronger antiseptics must be added; steam from hot water and vinegar inhaled into the lungs is harmless; this also helps expectoration, avoiding putrid corruption of the lung.

White sputa, and bland, light, even, odourless, of suitable consistency, are easily removed by coughing and hawking; they show that good pus is being made in the Ulcer; the Ulcer is now in a state from which it may recover; to ensure this, voluntary coughing to produce sputa should be restrained, and if the lung is irritable it may be quietened in the daytime by a draught of syr. de mecon., which will almost always quieten cough at night, ensuring that new vessels are not deprived of the protection of their own pus; now is the time for the most suitable nourishment: if good sputa are retained but the scanty and thick rejected, and symptoms relieved, the Ulcer heals very well indeed; if there is insufficient change the vessels of the Ulcer may be slightly occluded by suffitus gummi and a drier diet, both having been recommended.

In due course scarring takes place, recognised by cessation of sputum, quietening of cough and elimination of other ills; anything giving rise to Phthisis must be sedulously avoided, the lungs strengthened by equitation and other means and for a time the patient must keep to a strict diet.

All nourishment of Phthisical people must have these properties: similarity as far as possible to natural humours, coction being easy, that it be very nutritious, readily passing through the pulmonary vessels, and contrary to the disease. If the invalid has a warm temperament humours may be loose and acrid, veering easily towards decay; food must be ordered which is bland, acidmaking, but not stimulating, as prescribed for Haemoptysis; barley grain, prepared in the way stated, can be given at once; frequent use of this loosens the bowel too much, an inconvenience prevented by opium. Soup prepared from crabs, preferably river crabs and snails, is much esteemed. If tender meats and river fish are to be allowed, they must be cooked, or marinaded in acid. As a drink, milk and water, with a little sugar; or if a gentle and pleasing astringent is preferred, sweetened with conserve of red roses; if a spirituous drink is desired then moderately strong beer or canary wine are best, being nourishing; balsamics are also good, but do not combine well with milk; for producing a desired constriction a more austere wine may be preferred. But in a pituitous, cold state, beef broth is recommended, containing balsamic and aromatic herbs; a pinch of salt, orange or lemon juice may be added, or some Rhenish wine, for thwarting decay. The following serves very well as a drink: fresh egg, lightly cooked or raw, with sugar, shaken and diluted with milk and water; very tender broiled meat, with due seasoning, may be allowed at times; the choice of drink may lie between medicated beer and wine diluted with water, according to indications. All such may be allowed and varied according to the patient's temperament. If the patient is exercising, food should be prepared from pure sources, in small amounts and at such intervals that it is slowly mixed with the blood, and transferred easily to the lungs; avoiding hectic fever (if it threatens). If the first passages are too lax one can restore them with astringents. The invalid may avail himself of fresh air, travel and exercise as far as his strength allows.

Certain things must be sedulously avoided, for example: fat, glutinous, viscous and indigestible substances, but especially acrid and putrescent things: among these sugar & honey deserve special mention on account of their effect when large quantities are eaten; but I do not agree with Bennet that these putrefy on their own, for almost all acknowledge that they strengthen the humours; certain it is that when greatly weakened our humours tend towards decay and bad odour; which seems to happen with the daily consumption of mercury & scammony. Was this the reason, perhaps, that in acute fevers Hippocrates almost always added vinegar to honey?

If, after all, the inveterate disease harkens to no remedies, there is nothing left but for the physician to assuage the most troublesome symptoms; and so cough must be suppressed every night with narcotics; evening anxiety may be helped by light nourishment or calmed for a while by a drink of coffee sweetened with honey, or equally by a liquor aquoso tepido & incidente; dissolution of the blood by pus may be slowed by antiseptic substances; some have also tried to constrain them by astringents; white vitriol is especially commended, in a dose of $1-1^{1}/_{2}$ gr twice or thrice daily; liquid diarrhoea, which always occurs in inveterate Phthisis, killing the patient sooner or later, may be prevented by astringents, but more particularly by opiates; again if present it may be slowed down with the help of enemas, using theriac of Andromachus & Venetian terebinth, dissolved in white of egg & dilute milk; small quantities being repeatedly injected; by this means the most unhappy life of the patient may be preserved for a few days.

Notes

Thomas Glass's own references have been omitted throughout]

(1)   The word carina is used. This may be translated variously as the keel, the shell or in archaic anatomical terms the spine. Boerhaave himself speaks of 'the carina or incipient chick' in the English translation of his *Institutes of Medicine*, (London, 1742-1746), Vol.III, pp 346-355.   See also Nathaniel Highmore, *History of Generation*, (London,1651), pp 70-72.
(2)   Early anatomists, particularly Frederic Ruysch (1638-1731), outlined the vascular tree by injecting vessels with a coloured fluid which solidified on cooling. See D. Guthrie, *A History of Medicine*, (Nelson, 1958), p. 194.
(3)   Coction (concoction) is used in four distinct contexts; firstly as cooking, secondly as digestion. It is then used as a term for the physiological alteration to the chyle, so that as well as the digestive tract coction can take place in the absorbing vessels, the

lungs, and the blood. See Lester S. King, *The Medical World of the Eighteenth Century*, (Chicago,1958), p. 79. Lastly in the medical terminology of the time it signified the alteration made in the crude matter of a distemper, whereby it was either fitted for discharge or rendered harmless to the body. This could be brought about by nature, by the natural tendency of the matter itself or else by proper remedies. See R. Hooper, *Medical Dictionary* (London, 1831), p.399.

(4)   The primae viae are the stomach and small intestine, because they are the first passages of what is taken into the stomach; the lacteals are the secundae viae, because the nourishment next goes to them, and the blood vessels, supplied by the lacteals, the viae tertiae. Hooper, op.cit. p.1015.

(5)   Cacochymia. (From κακος, bad, and χυμος, juice or humour.) A diseased or unhealthy state of the humours. Hooper, op.cit. p.279.

(6)   Named after Sanctorius Sanctorius (1561-1636) of Padua, who made the distinction between beneficial invisible perspiration and sweating. D.Guthrie, op.cit., p. 197. For Boerhaave's views on the Sanctorian perspiration see op. cit. in Note (1) pp. 306-309.

(7)   Tabes. A term used in a generic sense for various wasting diseases, but distinct from phthisis, e.g. tabes mesenterica (the abdominal scrofula, of old writers), and diabetic tabes. Tabes dorsalis is used elsewhere in its correct sense as a form of advanced syphilis.

(8)   Distillation is a term used frequently in connection with the lungs, in the sense of a liquid dripping or trickling down and gathering in, for example, the bronchial tubes.

(9)   Revulsion (also known as derivation). A term used by the humoral pathologists, signifying a treatment by drawing humours a contrary way. See Hooper pp. 473, 1063. Galen, recommended the treatment of haemorrhage by opening a vein in another part. See P. Brain, *Galen on Bloodletting*, (Cambridge, 1986), pp. 12, 33.

(10) An issue, also known as a fonticulus is an artificial ulcer formed in any part by cutting a portion of the skin, and kept discharging by introducing daily a pea, covered with any digestive ointment. Hooper, op.cit. p. 592.

(11) Sal. polycrest (Polychrestus) or potass. sulphas, socalled because of its many virtues; a favourite with Boerhaave.

Rob. sambuc., the inspissated juice of the elder tree. Boerhaave gave its expressed juice in doses from a drachm to half an ounce, as a cathartic and hydragogue. It is said that whenever he passed an elder tree he raised his hat in acknowledgment of its therapeutic properties, but he is also reputed to have paid this compliment at the mention of the name of Sydenham.

(12) The Boerhaavian school made much of the six non-naturals in expelling or correcting hypothetical morbid matter. These were air, food and drink, motion and rest, passions of the mind, retenta and digesta, sleep and vigilance. See Lester S. King, op.cit. in note (3) p. 129.

(13) Decoction of the root of the common cinquefoil (Potentilla reptans). Hooper states that it was used by the ancients in the cure of intermittents but in the present day (1830) to stop diarrhoeas and other fluxes.

(14) Consolida= symphytum. Althea= marsh mallow (cum toto, both leaves and roots being used). Sem. lini.= linseed. Hordeum= barley.

(15) Suffumigra gummi, a resin burned to produce a pungent smoke or sweet smell when burned (suffumigation). Other substances used were mastich= pistachia lentiscus, the mastich tree, oliban= frankincense (thus), obtained from juniperus lycia,

styrax calamit. (officinalis) is a tree from which storax is obtained; sarcocolla is an exudation from a coniferous tree found in Persia, so named for its supposed property in gluing together the edges of wounds. Succinum= amber.
Hooper op. cit. pp. 1169, 977, 744, 1166, 1092, 1168.
(16) Τυλαιπωρεω, suffer from excess bodily toil, as with hard military service (hence misery).
πονος, work, labour. Also toil, trouble, fatigue, weariness, exhaustion, pain, distress, misery, sickness.
(17) Soaplike substances. See Hooper op. cit. p. 1089. 'With Boerhaave soap was a general medicine; for as he attributed most diseases to viscidity of the fluids, he and most of the Boerhaavian school prescribed it in conjunction with different resinous and other substances...'
(18) Hiera picra= Holy bitter; aloetic powder made into an electuary with honey. Hooper op. cit. p. 669.
Theriac. For a detailed account see G.Watson, *Theriac and Mithridatium* (London, 1960). Diatesseron of Mesue. A medicine compounded of four simple ingredients. Mesue was one of the early physicians among the Arabians. G.Watson, Ibid., pp. 125, 126.
Rheum= rhubarb. Fructus myrobalan, a dried fruit of the plum kind, brought from the East Indies.
(19) Cichoraceis= chicory (succory). Lignis sassafras= sassafras wood. Trium santalor.= sandalwood.
(20) Lapis haematites, bloodstone. This stone of a red colour has a long tradition in medicine for stopping haemorrhage; clearly an example of the doctrine of signatures and Frazer's 'homoeopathic' form of sympathetic magic. See Sir J.G. Frazer, *The Golden Bough* (Abridged edition, Macmillan, 1949), p. 12. Other red earths to which the same comment applies are bolus armena and terra lemnia (from Lemnos). Some earths were made into small flat cakes and stamped with a seal, hence *terra sigillata*.
Sanguis draconis= the dragon's blood plant (calamus rotang). So named for the red resinous juice, used in the same way. See Hooper op. cit. p. 282.
(21) The use of "S.M." as an abbreviation is enigmatic. It is suggested that it could be shorthand for Syrup de Meconio (syrup of poppies); opiates, then as now, a favourite remedy for consumption.
(22) "V.S." would seem to be an abbreviation of venesection.
(23) Balsamica. Substances of a smooth or oily consistency, possessing emollient, sweet, and aromatic qualities.
Incidentia. Medicines which consist of pointed or sharp particles, as do acids and most salts, which are said to 'cut the phlegm'.
Aromatica. Odoriferous or strong and agreeable smelling plants. See Hooper op. cit. p.165.
(24) 'B.L.', probably shorthand for *bene legendum*, indicating the passage is to be reread.
(25) Auripigmentum = yellow orpiment or sulphurised arsenic. So called for its gold colour and use to painters.
Sandaracha. Hooper mentions two forms, a gummy resin, and a form of arsenic. Sandaracha arabum is a resinous juice obtained from a large species of juniper tree. Sandarach or gum juniper was obtained from juniperus communis. Op. cit. pp. 214, 744, 1087.

Family tree (genealogical chart):

John Glasse = Elizabeth
d.1625   d. 1635

Peter d. 1651

Michael Glass d.1705

Thomas d. 1736

Sir Nathaniel Hodges = Mary Buttall   Thomas
d.1727   d. 1744

Michael = Elizabeth Handford   Mary   Michael   Peter   Elizabeth
1685-1732   1688-1770

Samuel Surgeon of Oxford

Robert
Thomas d.1780

Mary Hodges = THOMAS GLASS MD   Ann = John Lowder
1715-1783   1709-1786   1749-1821 1738-1810

Elizabeth
1742-1780

Melanie = Samuel Daniell
(Melony)
1751-1836

John Vowler Parminter = Mary   Dr Samuel Black   Elizabeth = Jacob Melhuish
                        1738-1776   d.1842   Surgeon of Tiverton

Rebecca   Anna   Charlotte

John Architect of Bath

Elizabeth   William

Charles = Sarah Fuge

Maria Glass
1762-1831

Thomas Glass
(Lowder)

Mary Ann = John Lees

Mellina   Charlotte   John   Dr Glass (Black)   Thomas Lees = Annie Taylor

John Lewis = Elizabeth Moffett

Charlotte   Mellina   John

see over

see over

see over

179

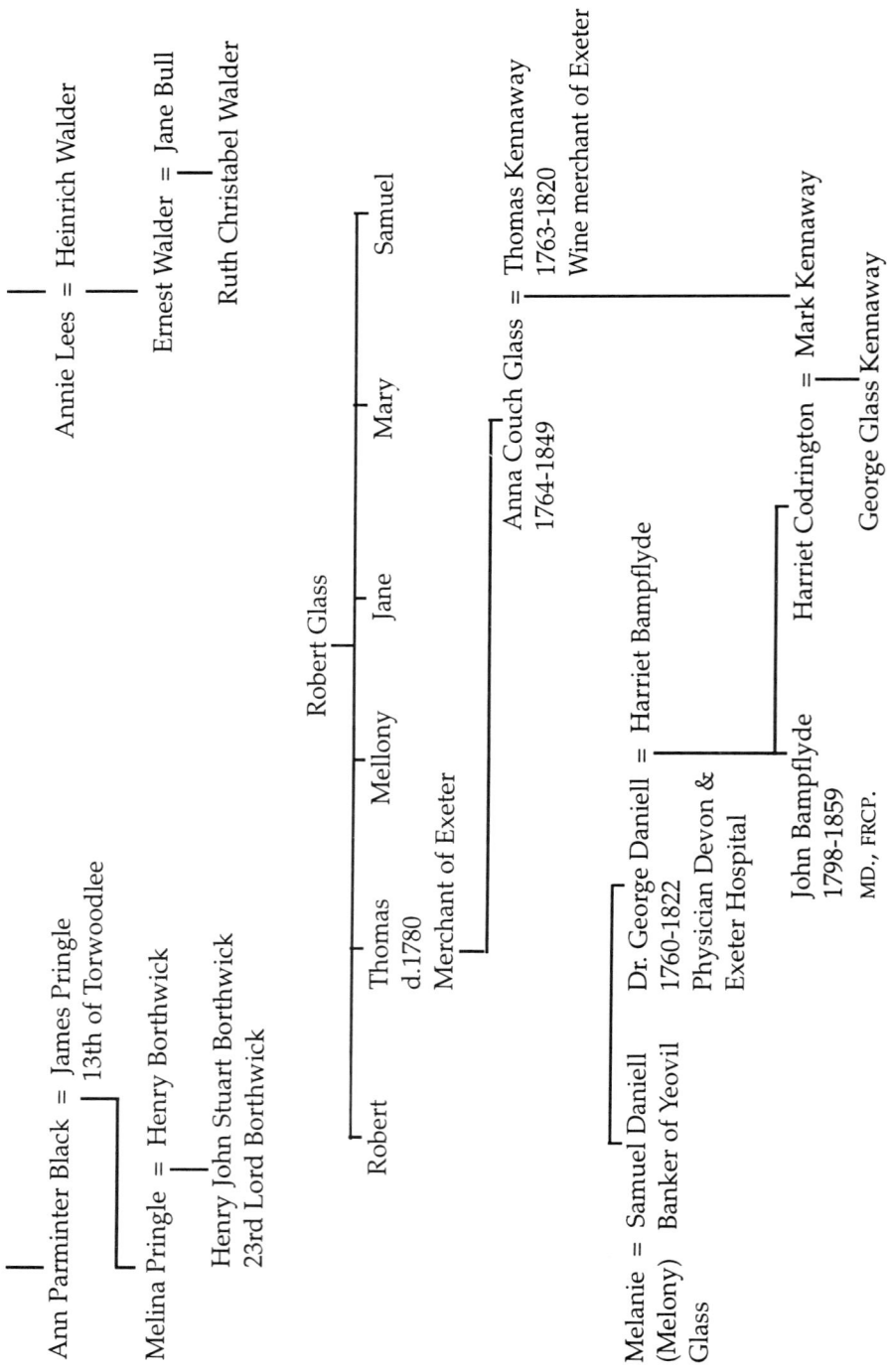

Annie Lees = Heinrich Walder

Ernest Walder = Jane Bull

Ruth Christabel Walder

Ann Parminter Black = James Pringle 13th of Torwoodlee

Melina Pringle = Henry Borthwick

Henry John Stuart Borthwick 23rd Lord Borthwick

Robert Glass

Robert — Thomas d.1780 Merchant of Exeter — Mellony — Jane — Mary — Samuel

Anna Couch Glass 1764-1849 = Thomas Kennaway 1763-1820 Wine merchant of Exeter

Melanie = Samuel Daniell (Melony) Banker of Yeovil Glass

Dr. George Daniell 1760-1822 Physician Devon & Exeter Hospital = Harriet Bampflyde

John Bampflyde 1798-1859 MD., FRCP.

Harriet Codrington = Mark Kennaway

George Glass Kennaway

180

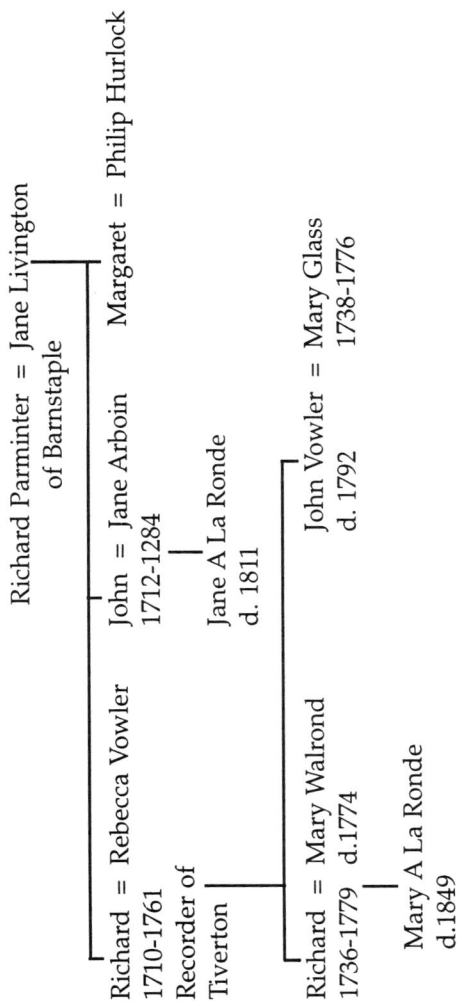

Richard Parminter = Jane Livingston
of Barnstaple

Richard = Rebecca Vowler
1710-1761
Recorder of
Tiverton

John = Jane Arboin
1712-1284

Jane A La Ronde
d. 1811

Margaret = Philip Hurlock

Richard = Mary Walrond
1736-1779   d.1774

Mary A La Ronde
d.1849

John Vowler = Mary Glass
d. 1792   1738-1776

Index

Glass, Elizabeth 20, 29, 38, 88-89, 91, 115, 135, 139-142, 179
Glass, Thomas 14, 17, 21, 27, 29-34, 38-40, 42, 48, 54, 57, 59, 61, 67, 81-82, 84-86, 90-91, 95, 98-100, 109-110, 112, 114-116, 122-124, 128-129, 131, 133, 135, 140-141, 143, 145, 176, 179
Glass, Mary (née Hodges) 11, 17-18, 21, 23, 29, 31-32, 136-143, 179-181
Glass, Michael 11, 17, 19, 29, 91, 179
Glass, Samuel 78-85, 87-94, 109
Glass, Thomas (senior) 17, 135-139, 179
Gregory, John 43

haemoptysis 127, 152, 154, 158-161, 164-168, 170-171, 175
Hamilton, Sir Alexander 138
Handford, Elizabeth 29, 135, 179
Hancock, Dr 54
Harris, J. Delpratt 15, 30, 44, 95, 107, 115, 128, 133-134
Harvey, William 67, 121
Haygarth, John 86
Heath, Benjamin 24, 27, 31, 39, 42, 44-45, 100, 140
Heath, Rose Marie 31
Heath, Thomas 27, 39-40
Heberden, William 12, 52
Henry, Thomas 79-80, 84-86
Hertford, Lord 102, 104
High Street, Oxford 87, 89-92
Hippocrates 9, 14-15, 20, 44, 58-59, 63-65, 67-68, 70-71, 76, 119, 126, 128, 151-152, 154-156, 158-161, 170-172, 176
Hodges, George 136-138, 143
Hodges, Lady Mary 17, 136-138, 143
Hodges, Mary (see Glass, Mary)
Hodges, Sir Nathaniel 11, 17, 29, 136, 137, 139, 179
Hoffmann, Friedrich 20, 44, 59, 76, 79
Hole, Richard 41, 107
Hole, William 41
Holloway, Richard 89
Hook, Dr 126, 146
horseriding 158
Hospital for Inoculating Poor Persons 55
hot and cold water baths 130
Houlton, Robert 48, 55
Hunter, William 108, 116
Huxham, John 11-12, 15, 47, 59-61, 69, 76-77, 82, 101-102, 106, 119, 128, 131, 134

Inaugural Dissertation at Leyden

124, 129
influenza 7, 14, 116, 118-119, 128
inoculation 7, 13-15, 21-22, 30, 46-52, 54-57

Jarcho, Saul 76
Johnson, Daniel 111
Johnson, Elizabeth 110
Johnson, Dr Samuel 12, 40, 104, 113
Johnson, Samuel 110-112

Leeuwenhoek, Anton van 60
'lentor' 15, 59-60, 70-73, 133
Leyden 7, 10-11, 15, 17, 19, 21, 29, 58, 87, 99-101, 108, 115-116, 123-129, 135, 145
Lind, James 12
Literary Society of Exeter 16, 38, 107
Llwythlan, Evan David 55, 57
London 11, 15-16, 29-30, 38, 40, 44-46, 49, 52, 57-58, 63, 76-77, 85-86, 91, 97, 99-101, 104, 107-108, 110, 114-117, 120, 123, 128-129, 134, 143-144, 176-178
Lowder, John 115, 140, 179
Lowder, John (junior) 140
Lowder, Lancelot 115
Luscombe William 142

Magnesia Alba 14, 78-79, 84-85, 88
malaria 63
malformation of the lungs 153, 167
Malpighi, Marcello 126, 146, 154
Mann, Sir Horace 29, 97
marasmus 151
Marchmont, Lord 114-115
May, Dr Nicholas 12, 13, 56, 57, 100
Mead, Dr Richard 59, 72, 76-77, 87, 92, 100, 107, 124, 132, 134
measles 76, 100, 121-122
medical 'systems' 14
medical ethics 43, 86
Medical Observations and Enquiries 116
Medical Society of Exeter 98
Meditations upon the Attributes of God 14, 42
miliary eruptions 37, 70
miliary fever 13, 19, 69, 72, 77, 110, 115
Moore, Rev. John 17
Mudge, John 41, 115
Mudge,Thomas 40
Mudge, Rev. Zachariah 40
Munk, William 12, 21, 29-30, 58, 76, 95, 101, 107, 143-144
Musgrave Samuel 15, 101-107

Musgrave, William 15, 101, 107, 133

nourishment 65, 145-148, 151, 157, 159, 164, 171-172, 175-177

Opie, John 15-16
Oliver, George 30, 95, 107
Oliver, William 11, 15, 42, 133
Oriel College 10, 58, 88, 92
Orme, Robert 138
Oxford 7, 10, 21, 25, 30, 40, 42, 58, 78-81, 84, 86-92, 101-104, 108, 116, 123, 179
Oxford Prison 87

Parminter, Jane 139-140, 181
Parminter, John Vowler 88, 139-141, 181
Parminter, Mary 115, 139-141, 181
Parr, Bartholemew (junior) 14, 20-21, 25, 27, 29, 31, 34, 39, 41, 44-45, 106, 107, 121, 122, 124, 126, 135, 140, 143
Parr, Bartholemew (senior) 31
Parr, Maria 39
Patch, John (junior) 96-97
Patch, John (senior) 95, 101
Patch, Robert 98
Patch, Thomas 97
Parker, Sackville 91
Percival, Thomas 12, 43, 80, 83-84, 86
petechial fever 73, 77
Peter Street 17
Peters, Nicholas 11, 22, 58, 78, 87, 109
phthisis 29, 115, 124, 127, 145, 152-154, 156, 159, 167, 169-172, 175-177
Pitfield, William 22, 30, 142
plague 72, 84, 120, 166, 171
plethora 150, 158, 165, 167-168
Plymouth 15, 17, 29, 40-41, 56, 59, 82, 100, 102, 104, 110-112, 115, 119, 121
Polwarth, Lord 113-114
Polwhele, Richard 12, 16, 38, 44, 107-108, 143-144
priapism 74
Prince of Wales 79
Pringle, Sir John 12, 15, 20, 77, 180
pulse 8, 52-53, 66, 70, 74-75, 109, 111, 126, 151, 165, 170
Pulteney, Dr 50
purgation 63, 155
purging 47-48, 53, 67-68, 70, 73, 109, 118, 130, 150
Pythagorick Numbers 63, 76

183